Breastfeeding, Take Two

successful breastfeeding the second time around

Breastfeeding, Take Two

successful breastfeeding the
second time around

Stephanie Casemore

GRAY LION PUBLISHING
Napanee, Ontario, Canada

Breastfeeding, Take Two:
Successful Breastfeeding the Second Time Around
by Stephanie Casemore

Gray Lion Publishing
282 Barrett Blvd.
Napanee, Ontario, Canada K7R 1G8

Printed in United States of America

Library and Archives Canada Cataloguing in Publication

Casemore, Stephanie, 1971-
     Breastfeeding, take two : successful breastfeeding the second time around / Stephanie Casemore.
Includes bibliographical references and index.
ISBN 978-0-9736142-1-3
     1. Breastfeeding--Popular works. I. Title.
RJ216.C343 2012   649'.33   C2011-904688-1

Editing by Sharon Dewey Hetke
Cover design by Diane McIntosh, Bright Ideas

The information presented in this book is based on the personal experience of the author. If you require medical or other expert assistance, you should seek the services of a competent professional. Before taking any course of action that may affect you, or your baby, it is strongly advised that you consult with a medical professional.

To Graeme, for enlightening me,
and
Elizabeth, for healing me.

With Love.

—Mom

Table of Contents

Skin-to-Skin Contact • Mothering from a Biological Perspective
• Importance of Mother's Health

Introduction

This book ultimately has a theme of finding balance. We all seek to find balance in our lives and work and family, but there is a deeper balance—a harmony that we yearn to find within our very being. This harmony isn't about fitting into the limited hours of the day the many responsibilities we all have or being able to cope with the challenges life throws at us on a daily basis. Instead, it's about reaching the balance that our very nature searches for. As both biological and social beings, there is a balance we must find between these often competing influences. We cannot give up our biological nature, nor can we live outside of social influences; instead it is necessary to find a comfortable middle ground where we can exist—to reconcile both our biology and our society. When we achieve a comfortable balance between the two, we feel more at peace.

Within every human is a deep-seated desire—whether consciously recognized or not—to find a balance, a harmony. We all want this, I believe, although we don't always recognize that this is what we are searching for. In our lives as mothers, it is no different. We unconsciously yearn for balance because it's natural to us. It is what we are intended for and when surrendering to it, we find it to be a place of ease—although perhaps not always an easy place.

A beautiful piece of poetry by Rabindranath Tagore, an Indian philosopher and poet, speaks so emotionally about this internal drive of mothering. A mother is not merely created the moment a woman gives birth, but is, according to Tagore, a compilation of experiences and emotions from generations past, as well as her own life experiences:

> "Where did I come from?" the baby asked its mother. She answered, half-crying, half-laughing, and clasping the baby to her breast, "You were hidden in my heart as its desire, my darling. You were in the dolls of my childhood games. In all my hopes and my loves, in my life, in the life of my mother, and in her mother before her, you have lived. In the lap of the eternal spirit you have been nursed and nurtured for ages."

In such an eloquent manner, Tagore has shed light on the emotions that surround the experience of mothering and breast-feeding—and the reasons they matter so much.

In this book I promise you one thing: I will not sugar coat the subject. I will not lie to you and I will not say "it's okay, some-times it just doesn't work out." Undoubtedly, you've already been told that. And likely, you weren't happy with that answer. This is why you are still seeking and searching for information and support to help you breastfeed your next child. What I hope I successfully do in this book is to shed light on the possible interventions of society and medicine that might have affected you and your efforts to breastfeed the first time around, and then give you information and advice for overcoming these influences on your second attempt.

The first half of the book focuses on these elements and how we, as mothers, relate to the breastfeeding experience, while the second half of the book provides more concrete knowledge and advice for creating a successful experience the second time around.

As new mothers we are confronted with a society that is far too concerned about not making a mother feel guilty or worrying that someone might feel pressured to breastfeed. But the common refrain of "It's okay to feed formula" or "Not everyone can breastfeed" isn't what we as mothers need. Of course if a woman has made an educated, informed decision not to breastfeed, then that's her prerogative. But too often women who want to breastfeed, who seek out support, simply don't get the support and accurate information they need.

Too often the support women receive is the equivalent of a marathon runner being told in the last mile of her race that it's okay to quit, she's tried hard, and that if she is tired and in pain, it's okay not to finish. Why are we saying this to people who have set their sights on a goal, prepared for that goal, but are experiencing difficulty achieving their goal? I don't want to provide that kind of support. I know I received that kind of support (and I know it was often well-meaning), but I believe when you've prepared for something and have set your sights on a specific goal, you should be supported and encouraged to *reach* that goal—not encouraged to quit—and only supported in a decision to stop once *you* have actually made the decision to quit the race. So in mile twenty-five of your marathon, I will be the one shouting, "You can do it", "You're almost there", and "You were meant to do this!" This is the support I needed and the kind of support I want to provide.

Too many moms today are traumatized. Often they have tried everything possible to successfully breastfeed their babies and still it doesn't work out. What's going wrong? Certainly this can't be nature's way. Humankind would never have managed to exist this long with the abysmal breastfeeding rates that we currently see. Yet mothers are told to accept it. Feed formula. Where did we get off track?

We've lost our balance—our harmony. Breastfeeding rates today are a symptom of our society's misfocus; we are a product of our society. But it is our responsibility and role to right ourselves when we discover imbalance—for the good of our children and our world, if not for ourselves.

This imbalance or lack of harmony is evident in our very primal experience of childbirth and breastfeeding. This imbalance not only affects us, more importantly it affects our children; this is why we need to do our part in recognizing it and trying to right the ship. This book is my effort to help right the ship.

Throughout the book you will read numerous personal stories from women, perhaps very much like yourself, who have struggled with breastfeeding. Some of these women have yet to try breastfeeding again with a new baby, some have found success the second time around, and some have tried again and still faced insurmountable challenges. The stories have been told in the women's own words and have been edited as little as possible. I felt it was important to have women share their own experiences in their own way without any limitations placed on them. For this reason, there is some inaccurate information presented in the personal stories, but these inaccuracies are in and of themselves important within the collective experience of women who are facing challenges breastfeeding: the information received isn't always accurate, the support isn't always ideal, and the influences of society are ever-present. Challenges come from many places and through the challenges these women faced, hopefully you will find inspiration, camaraderie, and support.

One of the most challenging aspects of writing this book was coming to terms with the concept of "breastfeeding failure". The connotations of the word "failure" are not ones I'm comfortable with, yet I have been unable to devise another term that can succinctly and easily express the idea of having not reached your desired breastfeeding outcomes. So for this reason alone, I have chosen to use the term "breastfeeding failure" throughout the book when necessary.

However, having looked at the subject from every angle, I've come to one conclusion: there is no such thing as breastfeeding failure. In truth, the only differentiation that is valid is "did" and "did not". The reasons for not meeting your breastfeeding goals are varied, but if you attempted to breastfeed — regardless of how long you actually breastfed — then you were a breastfeeding mom.

And yet many mothers will state that they failed at breast-feeding. If you are reading this book, chances are you were a mother who "failed" at breastfeeding. Who told you that you failed? Who or what determined your failure? These questions are critical to moving forward and breastfeeding successfully the second time around.

It took me a long time to realize that I didn't fail in my efforts to breastfeed my son. My experience certainly wasn't what I expected or hoped for, but I did breastfeed. I may not have ever exclusively breastfed my little boy without benefit of some type of supplementation device, and although I did exclusively pump for a year, he didn't nurse to any extent after he was about three months of age. I may have at times felt (and perhaps at times still feel) as though I could have done more to make it work. But in the end, I have realized that I was successful. I didn't have the experience I expected, but I did breastfeed.

The real issue is one of satisfaction. Success and failure is far too black and white for such a complex activity. You either did or did not breastfeed and within that black and white division there is a range of satisfaction.

If you are ultimately unsatisfied with your experience, then it is likely that you feel as though you didn't achieve success breastfeeding: you failed. But this ignores all you did do and the knowledge you gained—knowledge you will take with you to breastfeed the second time around. Life is merely an accumulation of experiences and growing in them is all we can hope to do. Even one day of nursing your newborn makes you a breastfeeding mom. Although it isn't likely what you intended and as a result therefore not a satisfying experience.

Now, let's move on from that experience and create a new opportunity; one that seeks to find balance and harmony and one that honours our biological nature while controlling the societal influences that may challenge our right to the breastfeeding experience we desire and expect.

Stephanie Casemore

July 2011

Sharon's Story

With my first pregnancy, I knew I wanted to breastfeed. My mother and sister both breastfed and a close friend was breastfeeding at the time. My sister had a good experience with her first child and a difficult time with her second, so I knew that some babies have latching difficulties. I had read books on breastfeeding and felt pretty confident about the basics. I was a little worried about the shape of my nipples being a problem, but I figured it would probably be fine.

I ended up having a lot of difficulty with getting my first baby to latch on. We went to three lactation consultants and I exclusively pumped for the first few months. We were then able to get him to nurse using a nipple shield. I was able to wean him from the shield around four months of age. Then we did a combination of nursing and formula when I went back to work when he was four months old. I was proud of the 250 ounces I had stockpiled in the freezer! He stopped nursing at nine months.

With my second pregnancy, I felt more confident in terms of the mechanics of nursing, pumping, and what to do if there was a problem. I was worried about having latching problems again. I was also worried I would again have to pump every few hours at the beginning, and I didn't know if I could do this with a two-year-old. I didn't think I would exclusively pump all of her milk—I would do a combination of breast milk and formula. As rewarding as it was to exclusively use breast milk with my first son, it was very time-consuming, stressful, and draining—literally! I was already concerned about being able to give attention to my older son and pumping would definitely interfere with this. I got everything ready for the possibility of having to pump and even brought my hand pump and some nipple shields to the hospital just in case.

With my first baby, I had been nervous and knew breastfeeding might be difficult, but it was much more difficult than I had expected. I was initially planning on nursing for one year, but a few weeks into it I thought I would be lucky to get to six months. I was also anxious about using my breasts for the purpose of feeding, as they had not been used in this capacity before.

With my second baby, I of course knew how difficult it could be. I planned on breastfeeding exclusively for the first four to six months then doing a combination because of having to return to work.

My second baby is six weeks old currently, and I plan on nursing up to a year. Although I can appreciate the beauty in breastfeeding, I am more the type that views it as the most healthy, natural, and inexpensive way to feed my baby. But I constantly think about how much easier it would be to use formula—especially in the first few months. I can see why many people just give up in the early weeks.

One reason I keep going is that I read that if you can just get through the first several weeks it is much easier. My husband is also very supportive and wants his children to receive breast milk because he views it as the healthiest diet for them. And not that I care too much about what others think, but most moms of middle to upper socio-economic status are expected to nurse (or at least try) nowadays and I do put this societal pressure on myself.

As for the breastfeeding experience specifically, with my first child he had latching issues from birth. We utilized the lactation consultants (LCs) and nurses at the hospital a lot. They set me up with a pump and I pumped small amounts of colostrum. I felt very disappointed about not being able to nurse and blamed myself. After all, it couldn't have anything to do with my perfect baby not being able to latch! We supplemented with formula under the advice of the hospital LC.

In the first few weeks, we used some formula and some pumped breast milk. Our goal was to use all breast milk and no formula, and this was achieved at around two weeks. We had a spreadsheet of how many ounces of formula/breast milk was given, diaper output, etc. I exclusively pumped for the first few months and then was able to nurse using a nipple shield. I remember being consumed by breastfeeding, scouring the internet and reading everything I could about the topic. I think this is one of the coping mechanisms certain people use in times of difficulty—researching to find as much information about a topic as possible.

The hospital LC department let me come back as an out-patient for more help and I believe this was instrumental in continuing to be able to pump and nurse with the shield. I also saw a private LC. She helped me to get the right sized flanges and pumping parts. She said that although he was latching, it was a dysfunctional latch and she was worried he wasn't going to be getting enough as he got older. She recommended cranio-sacral therapy to "fix" him and said he would have lifelong problems if I didn't do this therapy. Coming from a background of working with children with autism, I am very familiar with a wide range of holistic or alternative therapies and see families pay thousands of dollars with no results. I researched craniosacral therapy a great deal and did not find it to have any research or evidence to prove it to be effective.

This was a very difficult time for me, because I did not want to be seen as a bad parent who wouldn't do anything to help her child. But on the other hand, I did not want to spend hundreds of dollars for a therapy that is not proven to be effective.

Anyway, as my son got older, his latch got stronger. I think if we had been doing the craniosacral therapy it would have received the credit when really maturation helps a lot of these babies get stronger latches. Maybe it was just the way this LC said it when she suggested it, but this was one of the low points for me.

Using the nipple shield was exciting at first because he was actually latching on, but it became very cumbersome to keep it clean and ready, especially in the middle of the night. I was very excited when we started weaning from the shield. Then I returned to work when he was around four months old (I am a Speech-Language Pathologist working in a public school and I had the summer off). I only pumped once per day at work. I work with kids with moderate to severe autism and it put a strain on my co-workers for me to take off more time than that (even though they were supportive of my pumping at work). Also, I only worked seven-hour days and lived close to my son's daycare, so it wasn't too bad. I had stockpiled about 250 ounces so between that and pumping at work, I was able to use all breast milk up to six months of age. Then I did a combination of breast milk and some formula (and starting solids). At this point,

I was not as worried about the breastfeeding. I was happy that he was nursing in the mornings and evenings and did not stress about it as much.

At around nine months of age, my son started resisting the breast. I know I could have worked to get through the nursing strike, but I felt at peace that we were done nursing. I was also sick of being constantly rejected when I offered the breast. I missed nursing, but was also glad to be done. I felt very proud of myself for sticking with it. Why did I stick with it? We knew that breast milk was the healthiest and most natural diet. Also, I think my temperament of being a "type A" personality drove me to do a lot of research on pumping. I also had a great support system (my husband, family, and friends) who kept me going.

My second baby (a daughter) had a great latch from birth. I still constantly asked the LCs and nurses about the latch and they reassured me it was going well. She became really sleepy the second and third day of life. Although I had been told not to worry about the sleepiness, I was very worried especially when at one point she went four hours between feedings. My husband was home with our son, and I was alone with her at 2 a.m. trying to nurse for forty-five minutes. I finally buzzed for a nurse and burst into tears asking for help. They calmed me down and set me up with a pump I had requested. Since she was slightly jaundiced, they recommended giving her some formula and trying again the next morning after getting some rest. I was very upset but thought maybe the next day would be better. I felt better that I could pump colostrum for her. I remember it was more than what I was able to pump at the hospital with my first baby.

Then when we got home from the hospital we were able to nurse for most of the feedings. I still had to give some bottles of expressed breast milk because I didn't feel like it was working. She would shake her head around at the breast and just didn't get a good latch going. The LC helped me fine-tune some of the mechanics of nursing on the last day and this did help. I was not as confident because of the previous difficulties I had had. Now looking back, a lot of it was probably just normal "getting to know your baby" kind of difficulty. I pumped at the first sight of anything not going perfectly. I got easily frustrated and this probably made things worse. I was upset when my mom kept giving me the same advice over and over.

Then when I got engorged it was even worse! I didn't get as engorged with my first baby—I think maybe because I pumped exclusively with him that early on. Anyway, she couldn't latch at all to my engorged breast. I tried all the tricks such as pumping a few minutes before nursing, but it was so frustrating and painful! For those few days, most of the feedings were pumped breast milk. Finally when the engorgement went away, we were getting closer and closer to most feedings being at the breast. And that's where we are now.

She is six weeks old and getting almost all feedings at the breast, with occasional bottles of expressed milk when we have visitors or go out to eat, etc. I like having the freedom to use bottles sometimes, and I think it is good she is currently able to use both. I am already using my previous knowledge of pumping to help build my milk supply and work on my freezer stash—I already have 100 ounces stored. For awhile she constantly wanted to nurse and people would ask if I thought she was getting enough milk. This worried me a little, but she was having good output in diapers and I could see and hear milk transferring. She was in the 90th percentile for height and weight at her one-month check-up, so that put any concerns to rest! Now we are doing great and I am very grateful that she is able to latch.

There of course has been both short and long-term impact from my breastfeeding experiences. With my first baby, the short-term impact was additional stress, anxiety, and uncertainty. In the long-term, I think it taught me that motherhood isn't about being perfect. I am very proud of myself for sticking with it, but I wonder if I got too consumed with using my ability to provide breast milk to prove my worthiness as a mother. Looking back on the experience, I now know I would have still been a "good mother" even if I had had to give him formula.

With my second baby the immediate impact is that I am glad that I can nurse! I also feel validated that it wasn't "my fault" that I couldn't get a good latch with my first baby. Some babies have good latches and others have more trouble—it isn't always the mother's ability or not using a correct form to blame. Even though I was told this by the LCs I worked with, it still was amazing to me how much more easily my second baby was able to latch.

Breastfeeding is more difficult than many people realize. Most people think it's easy because it's so natural. But especially in the beginning, it can be very difficult for new mothers and babies to be successful at nursing. I have mixed feelings about nursing. Sometimes I really enjoy the bonding experience of nursing. Other times I see it as time-consuming and draining (physically and emotionally). Especially when my newborn wanted to comfort nurse or cluster feed and I was still sore, I thought many times how much easier formula would be. But in addition to the health benefits, there is still a drive in me to continue nursing as long as I can. It is the perfect food for my baby. I think although formula may seem more convenient, breast milk is still by far the better way to go. I would tell a new mom to try breastfeeding and keep in mind that the first few weeks to a month might be very difficult but after that things get much better. I would tell a struggling mom to try using LCs as resources and get as much information as you can, but if it doesn't work out she is not a "bad mom" for giving formula.

After I had the difficult experience with my first baby, I was nervous that the same thing was going to happen with my second baby. I did not think I would be able to devote the time to exclusively pumping with a two year old and a newborn. I wanted to make sure I was there for them and not always hooked up to a pump. I also didn't want to spend all of my time worrying and having anxiety about nursing with this baby. For these reasons, I would probably have been more likely to supplement with formula if I would have had trouble nursing this baby. Luckily, things are going great with nursing my second baby. She is now eight weeks old and I plan on nursing for as long as I can, and as long as she wants to continue. My goal is to continue some degree of breastfeeding until she is at least one year old.

Breastfeeding, Take Two

Section One

Understanding the Experience

The Great Balancing Act

"So much of how I view myself as a mother is tied to nursing."
Caroline, mother of four

B reastfeeding. Just the word can cause an emotional response in many women. Bring the topic up in a group of mothers and a great divide is often created between those who did and those who didn't, and in a very separate camp are those who desperately wanted to but couldn't or for whom it just didn't work out as hoped. Why is breastfeeding so emotionally charged? Why does it matter so much to us as mothers? The reasons why may not always be clear, but for those of us who have had a less than perfect breastfeeding experience, it is clear that breastfeeding is something deeply ingrained in our drive to mother. It is a desire that comes from within, and even though intellectually we understand that breastfeeding isn't always easy and isn't always possible, still it is something that many new moms yearn for.

To make matters worse, our society is often at odds with a mother's innate desire to breastfeed. Baby formula companies aren't shy about marketing to expectant and new mothers, often claiming that their products are "close to mother's milk" or contain elements found in mother's milk. A walk through any department store will lead you to long aisles filled with gadgets and devices intended to "make breastfeeding easier" — which of course is to suggest that it is difficult. Mothers are frequently in the news after being harassed for breastfeeding their babies in public. And while some countries are better than others at providing maternity leave for new mothers, many moms still need to head back to work after a few short weeks with their babies in order to maintain employment and pay the bills. It's no wonder breastfeeding is seen as being difficult and emotions are high.

When breastfeeding our babies is something that we expect to do, something we expect just to happen—it is natural after all, right?—but it doesn't work out as planned, we are often surprised at just how hard it is to let go of the dream, the expectation. Surprised by how emotional we become during the fight to make it work. Surprised at our determination to keep going—and our devastation when we finally decide to stop. You may have been surrounded by friends and family telling you just to quit and feed your baby formula and yet you wanted, even needed, to keep trying. You may have sought help and advice from anyone who would listen including doctors, nurses, lactation consultants, family, and friends. You likely cried many tears and perhaps endured some pain to try to make it work. And eventually you had to give up fighting, for the good of your baby, yourself, and your family; a mom's health and sanity are important to everyone, after all. Eventually, you arrive at a breaking point where something has to give, and so you quit breastfeeding.

But for many, this doesn't really make the experience any easier. Many moms who expected to breastfeed but found things didn't work out as planned have found they feel a great deal of guilt when they decide to wean early. Women then struggle, often for months or years, with the emotions swirling around in their heads and hearts. As I'll discuss later, I think guilt is often misnamed, and in fact what is truly being felt is grief, but with the official slogan of "breast is best" and the emotional debate that often surrounds breastfeeding, guilt is what most women will tell you they are feeling. But why? Why do we feel such an emotional reaction to breastfeeding—and not breastfeeding?

This chapter will delve into these questions and examine why we as mothers find breastfeeding to be such an emotional experience; we will consider the importance of breastfeeding within the continuum of pregnancy, birth, and the first few years of life; we'll explore how our bodies work to create an emotional attachment to our babies through the act of breastfeeding; and discover why the choice not to breastfeed or early weaning can impact our emotional state as new mothers, including increasing the risk of post-partum depression. Let's start though with the reason we, as humans, breastfeed in the first place.

Mammals After All

My son is nearing the end of grade two and he is now learning all about mammals. We all learned this information once upon a time, but with the lack of support and understanding of breast-feeding in our society, it seems as though it is something we all forget once we leave school: a cultural amnesia of sorts.

Mammals have several identifying qualities. The basic charac-teristics of mammals are that they have backbones, are warm blooded, give birth to live young, have hair, and have mammary glands. It is the last point which is most important to the discus-sion at hand. After all, if you have mammary glands they are there for a reason, no? In the mother, mammary glands produce milk and that milk is intended as nourishment for her babies.

While all mammals produce milk, the milk of individual spe-cies can vary widely depending on the needs of that particular animal. Specifically, the percentage of fat and protein varies depending on the environment and the parenting and hunting habits of the species. The milk of mothers who keep their babies close and nurse frequently throughout the day has a lower amount of protein than does the milk of species that leave their babies for long periods in order to hunt or forage for food. Mammals that require large layers of fat to protect them from harsh climates have higher amounts of fat in their milk. The composition of milk is also related to the growth rate of the species. Higher protein content ensures quicker maturation

The key here is that human females have breasts for a biological reason; that reason is the production of milk to feed their babies. So when trying to understand just why breastfeeding is such an emotional topic and experience, it is important to realize that we are dealing with biology—a biology that has a very lengthy history. For thousands and thousands of years, human mothers have put their babies to the breast to nurse and nurture. There was no question about the feeding method. That was it. If a mother was unable to feed her own baby, another lactating woman would step in or, as in more recent times, a wet nurse would be employed. There was no influence from advertising and big business to suggest women use other means of nourishment for their babies. Society and culture supported breastfeeding as it was intended: as the sole means of nutrition for infants with continued breastfeeding after the introduction of complementary foods until the age of weaning.

Of course if breast milk was not available, or an infant was unable to nurse, then a baby would in many cases die. This would have been a very harsh reality in times past. Fortunately in our modern society, we have the ability to provide alternative sources of nutrition that can nourish and sustain a baby quite well. Infant formula, or artificial baby milk, is a lifesaving substance that most definitely has its place in the appropriate circumstances. But unfortunately, all too often, formula is seen today as being on par with breast milk, which just isn't the case. Breast milk will never be matched, although formula companies continue to try. The business of artificial baby milk is just that—

business. Its goal is to sell product through marketing and advertising, not to ensure accurate and unbiased information is presented so that new mothers can make fully informed decisions. If you've never done so before, take some time to critically examine the intricacies and details of infant formula campaigns. The recent introduction of chocolate toddler formula should be an indication that formula manufacturers are not in business for the interests of our children!

Weaning, biologically, is also very different than the weaning that often takes place in our current society. Katherine Dettwyler, an anthropologist, has written extensively about breastfeeding and weaning from a cultural perspective. Through her research, she has estimated that a natural age for human babies to wean would be between two and a half to seven years of age.[1] This range is an enormous distance from what our society currently experiences given that some research suggests as few as fifteen percent of babies are exclusively breastfed at six months of age.[2] Cultural influences and society, again, affect our beliefs and actions with regards to weaning. Dettwyler says that she became interested in researching the natural age of weaning in part after realizing that other animals have consistent ages of weaning and that "presumably these animals don't have cultural beliefs about when it would be appropriate"[3] to wean.

So breastfeeding is biological. But culture and society has a great influence on our motives and beliefs making it more and more challenging to follow our biology. Yet understanding this division between our biology and society greatly informs the difficulty we have breastfeeding and the emotional state we find ourselves in when breastfeeding does not work out as expected. We are told that breastfeeding is natural and normal and that "breast is best". Yet, in many ways, society suggests actions that go against this natural and normal act. Mothers are caught in between these enormous weights: we have an inner drive to follow our biology but an outward pressure to conform to our culture and society. The official message being sent by pro-breastfeeding organizations and medical researchers constantly touts the "breast is best" message, but there is an equally powerful message coming from society at large suggesting that breastfeeding is not important and formula is the better way to feed your baby. Caroline, part of society but also feeling the biological nature of breastfeeding, shares this connection to breastfeeding when she says, "So much of how I view myself as a mother is tied to nursing. It doesn't make any sense." With this strong biological connection to breastfeeding and the conflict with society's attitudes towards breastfeeding, it's no wonder mothers feel confused, lost, frustrated, and guilty when it comes to breastfeeding challenges, and when breastfeeding doesn't work out.

Breastfeeding in the Continuum

One of the most influential books I have read over the past few years is *The Continuum Concept* by Jean Liedloff. While not a parenting book *per se*, Liedloff's book chronicles her experiences living with the Yequana people of South America and uses the lives of this group which was largely untouched by outside influences—and specifically the trappings of Western culture—to create a new vision of what human nature really is. Part of what she presents in her book is the concept of "the continuum" from conception through birth and infancy and into childhood and then adulthood. She suggests that we are born with biological expectations that have developed over generations and genera-tions of genetic evolution. Liedloff explains, "If one wants to know what is correct for any species, one must know the inher-ent expectations of that species." However, she goes on to explain that for those of us living in Western societies, under-standing what "evolutionary history has conditioned [us] to expect" can be difficult as "Intellect has taken over deciding what is best and insists on sovereignty for its vogues and guesses."[4] Our expectations for how we should be treated, and how we should treat others, come not so much from our understanding of our biologically inherent expectations, but from the societies and cultures in which we live. It is this division that has the potential to create many problems when it comes to breastfeeding.

Liedloff discusses numerous aspects of biological expectations including the expectations a baby has after it is born. Breastfeeding is included among them. And this points to another reason why we as mothers find breastfeeding to be such an emotional experience. Imagine thousands and thousands of years of evolution and genetics culminating in the birth of your child and then society interferes with its lack of support for breastfeeding; its insistence that mothers return to work often within weeks of giving birth; its pressure that feeding should be considered a method of bonding for not just the mother but for the father, siblings, and extended family; its view of a woman's breasts as sexual objects resulting in her feeling uncomfortable about using them for any other purpose; and its requirement that a mother should encourage—demand—a baby become independent of her at almost the moment of birth. With all of this taken into consideration, it is amazing that babies are still breastfeeding. Yet nature is amazing in its persistence and determination, and our babies are born with the reflexes and skills in place that allow them to breastfeed.

Honouring Nature

While it might seem to be a bit of a tangent, the words of Cesar Millan, the Dog Whisperer, strike me as particularly applicable to the discussion of breastfeeding and biology. Although Millan works with dogs, what he is really applying to his work is the idea of balance with Mother Nature. In many ways, he is presenting a way of being that is very similar to what Jean Liedloff suggests is necessary. On one episode of *The Dog Whisperer* Millan states, "If we learn to honour what they need, we create balance." He is of course speaking of dogs, but the same is true for babies. We are dealing with nature and biology when we are nurturing our babies. Accepting and honouring our babies' needs will most definitely assist us in creating balance — for ourselves as well as our children. Millan's ideas are remarkably similar to Liedloff's and also follow similar principles to the work of Suzanne Colson among others who are striving to reconnect to the simple biological mechanisms that our culture has sought to push aside — and in reconnecting creating balance and a more natural way of being.

Birth, Bonding, and Breastfeeding

These inherent skills present at birth are in fact so strong and focused that a baby, if left to his or her own devices, can actually crawl from the mother's abdomen to the breast, locate the nipple, and latch on, all without any intervention from the mother.[5] This process is in fact an important first step in the bonding and imprinting that begins following delivery.

Birth, bonding, and breastfeeding are part of an important series of events that assist both mother and baby in developing a strong attachment to one another. Immediately following delivery, the mother's brain is flooded with oxytocin which is an amazing hormone. When breastfeeding, oxytocin is passed to the baby through the mother's milk; both mother and baby benefit from its effects. Known as the hormone of love, oxytocin serves many roles including eliciting the milk ejection response in breastfeeding women and contractions of the uterus during labour and childbirth, but one of its most important roles is in the development of love and attachment.

A study by Ruth Feldman, PhD, of Bar-Ilan University discovered that women with higher levels of oxytocin in the first trimester of pregnancy bonded better with their babies and that higher oxytocin levels throughout the pregnancy resulted in an increase in behaviours that assisted in the later development of strong relationships with their babies.[6] An animal study conducted by Karen Bales of the University of California indicated that oxytocin exposure early in life is connected to better maternal and social behaviours later in life.[7] The wonders of oxytocin are seemingly limitless and are certainly an important aspect of the process of bonding between a mother and baby.

It is important to mention that the synthetic form of oxytocin, pitocin, which is well known due to its use to induce labour and encourage contractions, does not cross the blood-brain barrier and therefore does not cause the same bonding response in new moms as does natural oxytocin. Mothers who receive pitocin may never benefit from the hormonal boost of love and maternal feelings oxytocin creates. This isn't to say moms who are induced will not bond with their babies, but they won't experience it in the same way.

The boost of oxytocin, and its bonding effects, is experienced every time a mother nurses her child. The oxytocin passes through the milk to the child increasing the effects. It is this knowledge which helps us understand, yet again, why breastfeeding is so emotional and why it means so much to us as mothers. Every time a mother nurses her baby, she gets that flush of oxytocin and the warm, relaxing feeling it brings. Her baby also experiences this and the connection between mom and baby is heightened and strengthened. Breastfeeding then, while not the only way to promote bonding, does make the process easier and creates a continuing flow of the "hormone of love" between a mom and her baby. Most breastfeeding moms talk about the closeness of breastfeeding and oxytocin has a lot to do with it.

Breastfeeding and Emotional Calm

If you've ever witnessed the blissed-out expression of a baby after breastfeeding, you have witnessed the wonderful calm and sense of peace that oxytocin can create. Research has shown that mothers who breastfeed are calmer under stress than their bottle-feeding counterparts.[8] In a review of research dealing with lactation and its impact on stress, Maureen Wimberly Groer et al. discuss the protection against stress that breastfeeding provides explaining that "This protection appears to be governed by the neuroendocrinology associated with lactation, which is the natural, biologic normative behavior of all postpartum animal mothers. This protection makes evolutionary sense in that the maternal-infant dyad is protected and supported by these responses."[9] Every new mother faces stress and emotional upheaval; it's a common experience among all new mothers as hormones are stabilizing and daily life is finding a new balance. Yet the fact that breastfeeding appears to ease the stresses of daily life may not be your experience if you've had difficulty breastfeeding. When we have become so distanced from our natural behaviour and limited in the amount of support we receive post-partum, the difficulties experienced in the early days of breastfeeding can in fact cause a great increase in stress. However, it is important to recognize that breastfeeding is the biologically normal state and balance that our bodies naturally yearn for and expect.

The cruel fact for those who have experienced breastfeeding difficulties is that what should be a time of relaxation, enjoyment, and rest ends up being a time of increased stress, pain or discomfort, and anxiety. Somewhere in the back of our minds we realize that this isn't how it should be, and I believe that we as new mothers are seeking the balance and calm that should be part of a new mother's experience. Our society has made it more challenging for moms to achieve this experience through breastfeeding due to a lack of social supports, the normalization of bottle-feeding, and the failure to pass breastfeeding knowledge along from one generation to the next. So we then seek to create this balance for ourselves, often by giving up on breastfeeding in an effort to resolve what we perceive as the cause of the stress and turmoil.

Yet, remember that it is our cultural and societal influences that are often at play when breastfeeding difficulties happen. While it may seem as though it is breastfeeding that caused you the greatest amount of stress in the early post-partum period, in reality it is the division between what is biologically expected and what is socially supported. Our biology wants us to breastfeed, wants our babies to breastfeed. We, as new mothers, want to find the harmony and calm that we know should exist with our new baby and this separation between biology and society is, again, one of the reasons why breastfeeding is so emotion-filled. We need to strive to reconcile these two ever-present forces.

Post-Partum Depression

Upon gathering from women their stories of breastfeeding "failure" to include in this book, I was struck by the fact that a number of women questioned whether their inability to breastfeed was indeed a cause, at least in part, of their post-partum depression. It is difficult to determine whether women wean early due to depression or whether early weaning contributes to depression. What is apparent is that while breastfeeding does not prevent all cases of post-partum depression, there is evidence showing that moms who breastfeed experience less depression.[10] Post-partum depression is unfortunately not that uncommon and many new moms do suffer from less serious "baby blues". The connection between depression and breastfeeding challenges may not be clear, but it is evident that both can cause a great deal of suffering for a new mom. Caroline, who had challenges nursing one of her babies and who suffered from severe depression, was told she could either nurse or take the medication needed. She opted for the medication but says, "I feel like I suffered just as much by feeling like a failure as a mother." The impact of breastfeeding difficulties and depression are equally devastating to mothers.

Alison Steube, a maternal-fetal medicine physician, notes in an article on the *Breastfeeding Medicine's* blog that "...there is ample data that social support, maternity practices, and other factors impact breastfeeding outcomes, and it's entirely possible that poor support leads to both depression and to early weaning."[11] Steube's insight again highlights the importance of both following and supporting our biologically driven expectations of motherhood.

How can we expect new mothers who have never seen a baby breastfeeding, never learned the normal feeding patterns of a newborn, and have never been taught sound breastfeeding practices during their pregnancy to easily breastfeed their babies? While breastfeeding is biologically driven, it must be socially supported. In order for mothers to experience the normal process of breastfeeding, it must be made normal in our society.

Our emotional ties to breastfeeding are strongly connected to our biological make-up. While we may not be consciously aware of these biological drives, they are there nonetheless. In understanding the emotions that are at play in our post-partum selves, we must view them through the lens of our biology and recognize just what we have, and do not have, control over.

The "Breast is Best" Buy-In

Over the past couple of decades, the struggle to increase breast-feeding rates has been championed by many, and this movement, like many movements, has a slogan. Everyone knows it. Everyone has heard it. Breast is best. The problem with this slogan isn't in its message. It is hard to disagree that indeed breastfeeding is best for babies. The concern with the "breast is best" message comes in its separation of mothers into two groups: those who breastfeed and those who don't. A better message would be "breast is normal".

Breastfeeding supporters, or lactivists, have done a wonderful job of sharing the message that breast milk is the best thing for a baby. However, absent from this campaign has been the implementation of social supports to assist new moms in achieving successful breastfeeding. Overwhelmingly, new mothers state their intentions and desires to breastfeed. Most areas boast statistics well in excess of 80% of new mothers who intend to breastfeed. Yet the figures for babies who are still receiving any breast milk at six months of age are dismal; and worse yet are the numbers of babies who are *exclusively* breastfed at six months. A recent report from the Centers for Disease Control in the United States indicates that while 75% of babies are breastfeed at some point, at three months of age only 33% are exclusively breastfed and at six months only 13.3% are exclusively breastfed.[12] In Canada, the statistics are similar with 87.5% of babies breastfeeding for some length of time, but only 24.4% are breastfeeding exclusively for six months or longer.[13] Why, when the "breast is best" campaign has become so ingrained in our society, are we still not seeing strong breastfeeding rates? Why are women still finding the path to breastfeeding fraught with difficulties? We have bought into the message, but we have not been given the skills necessary to achieve it.

So why does breastfeeding matter so much?

The answer is quite simply: because we are mammals and that's what we do. As much as our society tries to distance us from our basic biological instincts and functions, our biology still drives our actions and impulses. Mothers are biologically primed to nurture and care for their babies. Regardless of how our society distances us from our biology, there will never be a complete separation.

The gap between our societal practices and our biological drives can create a challenging problem for new mothers. Listening to our bodies, but fitting into our society, is often difficult. Our society suggests babies should sleep on their own, become independent early, learn to meet their own needs, and be able to thrive under multiple caregivers. Society also encourages women to return to work soon after the arrival of a new baby, share parenting responsibilities equally between parents, and limit the bonding between mother and baby to create the independence our little ones need in order to switch easily between caregivers. These things are all contrary to our biological drive to mother. Yet the fact of the matter is that for many mothers, the requirements of society are unavoidable. Income must be made to survive. This necessitates placing young babies into full-time childcare and having fathers participate equally in parenting. But the biological drive is still there.

In theory and in practice we must figure out how to reconcile these two forces: biology and society. Understanding the interplay between them will provide us with the ability both to make an informed choice and better understand the strong emotions we feel when it comes to mothering and breastfeeding.

Michelle's Story

I cannot say that I grew up with a very positive attitude toward breastfeeding. In reflecting on my pre-pregnancy stance more intentionally I see that a combination of early childhood experiences as well as a prejudice within my own family led me to marginalize breastfeeding, relegating it to that body of things I would probably never do or want to do. There are a few contributing factors to this sense of being an outsider, among them some pivotal events that left a lasting impression and that might have contributed to my eventual failure to breastfeed. At the very least, they help to explain why I gave up so quickly.

First and foremost is the fact that I was never breastfed myself. From an early age, I knew that my mother breastfed my sister but that she didn't have a chance to breastfeed me. I was put in the care of a babysitter in September of 1971, barely six weeks old, when my mom had to go back to her job as an elementary school teacher. As complex as my relationship with my mother has been in the thirty-eight years since my birth, I have often managed to distil all of our problems—particularly the lack of intimacy between us—down to the fact that she never truly bonded with me as an infant. In my mind, breastfeeding was a prerequisite for a genuine mother and child connection and I've always carried a good deal of sadness that we missed the opportunity. To make matters worse, and only serving to strengthen my case, is the fact that my mother and sister have a very special relationship, exhibiting a unique and visible bond, one which I attribute to the fact that she was breastfed and I was not.

The second contributing factor to my feelings of isolation is that I had a somewhat traumatic encounter with breastfeeding as a preschooler that, ironically enough, made me think of it as gross and unnatural. My mother ran a home daycare for a time and the mother of one of the children was a kind of stereotypical 1970s earth mother, bathed in tie-dye, the kind of woman who probably had sundials all over her living room and homemade yoghurt and bread in her kitchen. When she would come to pick up her son, the feeding frenzy would begin. The greedy little boy would grab at her loose flowing skirts and climb up to her belly and shout "tit, tit" and she would whip it out and he would latch on with fervour. I would look away, but the symphony of suckling was perhaps most unbearable of all. This was quite shocking to my four-year-old sensibilities and seemed totally foreign. My mother's reaction only reinforced my disgust, as after the two left she would shuffle around the kitchen, huffing and ranting that breastfeeding "at that boy's age" was "totally over the top".

Thirdly, and perhaps most significantly, was that in late adolescence I became cemented in the notion that women are actually divided into two distinct categories: those who are the "type" to breastfeed and those who are not, and that I belonged most definitely to the latter category. I was on an outing with my dad, accompanying him to visit the farm of one of his cousins. It was a typical northern Ontario dairy farm, with a typical farmer's house inhabited by a typical farmer's family. When we arrived, we smelled an odd combination of muddy boots caked with manure and freshly baked blueberry pie, and we were greeted by a timid young woman so heavily laden with children it was a feat of athleticism for her to move the ten feet from her kitchen stove to the back door to let us in. Toddlers encircled every available appendage of the poor woman's body. Most memorable for me was the plump babe with a ruddy complexion and tiny jam-soaked fingers, suspended from the teat of her mother's long floppy boob. To an aspiring cosmopolitan girl like me—desperate to escape the hell of northern Ontario for big city salvation—this was anything but an idyllic scene. I don't remember if it was the heroic display of motherhood or the thought of my breasts ever becoming that stretched out and gummed up with jam, but at the time I decided the whole thing was not for me.

As if to put an exclamation point on my silent but visible resolution, my father told me quite emphatically, as we drove away that day, that he could never imagine me ending up with "children all over my hips and boobs like that." He stated it with a measure of relief on my behalf, as if my aspirations—when fulfilled—would lead me down a much smoother path. As the years went by, I sadly took his comment further than was intended, thinking he couldn't imagine me being a mother at all, or that I wasn't the mothering type. My father died before my son was born and there have been many times that I wished he were alive to see that my finest life achievement has been the care and nurture of this amazing little boy that God has entrusted to me.

All this is to say that by the time I entered my twenties, breastfeeding was for other women and it was not something I thought about, not even in passing. That all changed, of course, in the summer of my thirty-fourth year, on the day I saw the little peanut of an embryo I thought I'd miscarried flickering on the screen of an ultrasound technician's monitor. That's when the next phase of my adventure in breastfeeding would begin.

During pregnancy my attitude toward breastfeeding evolved as if in sync with each trimester, having three distinct phases. The first phase was characterized by disbelief and wonder, the second by insight and awareness and the third and final phase was hope and conviction. It was an interesting journey that I remember well.

Having spent the majority of my first trimester either asleep or looking for places to sleep due to the ridiculous fatigue that set in, I don't remember a whole lot about those few months. But I do remember noticing for the first time that near my office was a branch of La Leche League. I would have walked by it many times; what did I think that was before I got pregnant? When the layers of things I needed to begin to think about started opening up for me, I felt a real sense of wonder and amazement that breastfeeding had become such an industry.

I was very surprised to learn that breastfeeding was difficult. I thought that if you wanted to do it you just did it and if you didn't want to do it, well, you just didn't. By the time I hit my thirties I had matured enough in my thinking to no longer view breastfeeding as gross and, in fact, it occurred to me that it would probably be about the most natural thing a person could do. The amount of advice and counselling one could get, the sheer numbers of contraptions one could invest in, the full gamut of the books that were available for sale came at me with a dizzying pace leaving me utterly bewildered. I thought it was supposed to be easy; that a person could "fail" to breastfeed or that one would need to learn to do it or be instructed in the art of it was an eye-opener indeed.

Once I got over the shock of that and once I made it through my first trimester after having had a couple of previous miscarriages, I tried to slow the wheel of information enough to hop on and start spinning. I spent the lion's share of my second trimester in the information gathering phase, trying to learn everything I could about this mystical, magical thing called breastfeeding. Even though I knew that the seeds of a positive outlook on this thing had not been sown in my early life, I was determined to give it a try. I chose a midwife as my primary health provider; I read the pamphlets; I believed in the science of this ultimately natural and supremely nutritious source of food for my baby. I loved the idea of being out and about and not having to mess around with bottles. I was terrified of formula and became quite vocal about it and managed to offend both my mother and my mother-in-law: "Well you were both [my husband too] formula babies and you were extremely healthy, thank you very much." But the more I read and the more I talked to other women about their experiences, the more anxious I became. So I added breast-feeding to the list of things I lost sleep over at night in advance of my son's birth. It didn't rank as high as my fear of an episiotomy or of losing control of my bowels in front of an entourage of medical students, but it was definitely high on the list.

As I moved into my third trimester, sensing that I was whip-ping myself into an unnecessary fit of panic and anxiety, I decided to try to let go. I was not particularly successful with this. But I put down my breastfeeding manuals and decided to just hope and pray that it would work out. In a way, I wanted to regress to the place I was before where it would be so natural and easy. My son would be born, I would hold him close to my breast and some mix of instinct and ancient wisdom buried deep within would take hold of me and magically affix my son's tiny mouth to my boob the way God intended. I did a lot of hoping and a lot of praying and at that point it was a much better strategy than doing any more researching and analyzing.

And then my son was born.

Let's see, how shall I characterize my breast-feeding experi-ence....I was introduced to breastfeeding by a kind-mannered, but very male nurse. With a burning pain in my abdomen from a c-section, a dizzying fog in my head from the general anaes-thetic, and an ache in my heart for not being able to crawl into my bed with my little boy, I didn't know whether to laugh or cry at the irony of a man teaching me how to breastfeed. All I could do was surrender to the process. Perfectly healthy, but just shy of the 5-lb benchmark that would have secured his release from the hospital, my son Joseph and I were in limbo until I could prove to the medical masses that I could successfully feed my baby.

In the middle of a cramped NICU full of people watching the clock, waiting for me to get the job done—watching, assessing, measuring whether or not I was up to the task of feeding my child—my two-week breastfeeding odyssey began. Gone, it seemed, was any concern for the mother and child union; the only thing that mattered was my ability to produce, or to "establish feeding" as I heard the doctors mumble as they made their daily rounds.

Like a twenty-first century Wonder Woman, armed with the plastic breast shield—the indispensable intermediary the nurses told me was the only hope for us—Joseph and I became part of the fabric of the NICU for ten days. After feeding, I would be politely nudged out of the NICU and would return to my dingy little "guest room" in the hospital, usually reserved for the families of out-of-town ICU patients. Every three hours like clockwork I would get a call from the nursing station asking me to come back and feed him again. Altogether it was a very clinical experience, one that I have only recently cleansed myself of. I felt like a miserable failure most days and it took me almost three months to gain any sense of confidence in my skills as a mother.

I went home completely petrified that I would starve this tiny boy and within forty-eight hours I asked my husband and my sister to go get some bottles and formula. There was a time in the hospital when I asked to put him on the bottle; it seemed logical to me since he was very small and maybe a bottle would be better for him. But I felt a sense of shame at the reaction of the nurses and my family members—don't give up so fast, they said. I just knew in my heart that it wasn't going to work. Maybe it was the lack of a cultural legacy around breastfeeding— absolutely that played into it—but I was exhausted from a challenging pregnancy and a stressful birth and I just wanted to feed my baby and take him home.

Joseph was so small and there was too much guesswork involved with determining the quantity of milk he would get from his feedings. He started to put on weight almost immediately when I switched to the bottle, and he drank and drank and drank like there was no end to his hunger. I felt relieved more than anything and it just felt good to feed him and hold him and to know that he was thriving.

Any anxiety I had about not breastfeeding and the impact it might have on my bond with my son completely faded away. I cannot imagine us being any closer or more connected than we are. If I have any lingering guilt or regret about anything, it was in not enjoying those first days with him—just holding him and feeding him—as much as possible. The bottle was a great option for him; he didn't have to struggle to take it and I didn't have to struggle to give it to him. I feel very sad that women have lost the ancient wisdom and the sisterhood that made breastfeeding easier. Although perhaps it is only my perception that it was easier, that it must certainly have been easier; maybe it has always been difficult.

I wish it had worked out for us, but I don't lament the fact that it didn't. When I see friends and other women who seem able to do it with ease, I truly celebrate for them and don't feel any sense of jealousy or inadequacy. When a friend tells me she is planning to breastfeed, I don't pipe in with my fifty cents worth of unwanted and unneeded advice and offer a slow and painful rewind of my difficult experience. Instead I say a silent prayer that the circumstances of her baby's birth will lead her to the outcome she seeks.

I am not planning on having another child now, but about a year ago I considered it very seriously and in the process of visualizing it, playing the movie forward in my head, the idea that I would try again to breastfeed was very much a part of that visualization. I cannot imagine if I had a healthy, robust baby and a less medicalized birth experience that didn't leave me so thinly stretched, that I wouldn't absolutely give it a try—and give it a try in earnest and with much greater privacy.

What's Society Got to Do With It?

"I feel very sad that women have lost the ancient wisdom and the sisterhood that made breastfeeding easier."

Michelle, mom of one

T he world around us—our society and culture—plays an important role in how we perceive breastfeeding. We learn about breastfeeding from our family, our friends, and more and more frequently, from the media. Breastfeeding, which at a base level is most definitely a biological process, is also a social behaviour. While we may as mothers have inherent instincts and abilities to nurture our infants, we learn how to breastfeed—and how to mother—from those around us. When these two forces collide, mothers are left confused and have to choose between acting on culture or acting on biology. Cynthia Good Mojab explains that "…breastfeeding problems are often rooted in cultural beliefs and practices that do not match the biologically based needs of mother and child. When new breastfeeding information challenges a mother's culturally based beliefs, she may mistrust it and have difficulty acting on it."[1] Being able to understand the cultural messages and balance them with the biological aspects of mothering is important, but can be challenging. It is vital that we, as women and mothers, consider these conflicting messages being transmitted to us and educate ourselves to make choices that are in the best interest of those involved—mother and baby.

The current debate surrounding breastfeeding is all about the choice between formula and breastfeeding. Which one is better? Can't parents make their own decisions about their babies' feeding? Why make moms feel guilty about something that they can't do? Is this debate different than what would have taken place a hundred years ago? Two hundred? Most certainly it is. There have always been babies who had difficulty breastfeeding and mothers who chose other feeding options. A baby with a cleft palate would likely not have survived and infants were often fed not by their mothers, but by wet nurses. This was normal and part of many societies. Certainly some societies offered various other supplements and foods to infants and sadly there was a significant mortality rate. Yet, for the most part, breastfeeding was still seen as the way to feed a baby; it just wasn't always mom doing the feeding.

But sometime over the past hundred or so years, breastfeeding has been derailed. An emerging modern view of science as an unquestioned vanguard of progress heralded in scientifically prepared formula as the better method of infant feeding. Prudish attitudes towards women's bodies and sexuality impacted the way society viewed birth and breastfeeding. Women's liberation meant women were no longer tied to maternal roles but could make choices that allowed them to be and do anything. And overriding it all was an advertising industry that learned they could influence the attitudes and values of society with carefully crafted campaigns aimed at their target market—advertising campaigns that all too often create a need instead of meeting one.

There is no doubt that infant formula, or artificial baby milk as it is sometimes called, is a life-saving invention. There are most definitely situations that require a safe, alternative infant feeding method. But while formula has gained in popularity and acceptance, it has done so to the detriment of breastfeeding. Unfortunately, while infant formula is big business and the companies that manufacture it push hard to capture their share of the market, there is no significant marketing budget for the advertising of breast milk.

This chapter looks at the current state of breastfeeding in popular society and invites you to consider and question the influences that shape *your* understanding of breastfeeding, the attitude of those around you, and the effect of these influences on your breastfeeding efforts. Whether we like it or not, we are social creatures and we are part of a cultural machine that includes strong influences particularly from media and advertising. It is perhaps foolish to think that these things do not influence our parenting—including our attitudes, ideas, and understanding of breastfeeding.

While you read through this chapter, I challenge you to question your own attitudes about parenting and breastfeeding. Where did they come from? Who or what helped to shape them? Are they positive or negative? Are they constructive or destructive? Do they support your biological ability to breastfeed or are they counterproductive to natural processes? This isn't about placing blame or looking for excuses. It's about seeing things for what they are and being able to move past where we are and towards where we want to be.

The Current Face of Breastfeeding

Breastfeeding has two distinct faces in the media. One would suggest that it's easy and everyone should do it. And the other offers an image of something that, while good for baby, is often difficult and painful, something to be endured. There are certainly truths to both sides of the story, but the reality mostly lies somewhere in between.

Our society has set up a dangerous expectation making mothers believe that breastfeeding is always a wonderful, enjoyable, lovely experience. It certainly is at times, but it isn't *always* wonderful. In *Unbuttoned*, a book containing essays examining both the pain and pleasures of breastfeeding, Julia Glass clearly states how many women expect to experience breastfeeding saying, "they assume the pain would end at childbirth and the joy would begin at the breast."[2] Laura, a mother who endured pain and numerous challenges in the effort to breastfeed her son thinks "breastfeeding is presented in an overly simplistic, idealized light—as though it's as simple as 'choosing' to breastfeed and 'hanging in there through the initial discomfort.'" This expectation that breastfeeding will be all love and cuddles can be just as devastating as the belief that breastfeeding will be painful and demanding. Clearly we need to find a middle ground.

I nursed my second child for three years, and there were certainly times that I couldn't stand the idea of continuing. But I did and I'm very glad I did. Problems can come and then they usually go. Just as with everything, there is good and bad. Enjoy the good and try to minimize the bad. Ultimately, breastfeeding is about providing the biologically normal form of nourishment for your baby via a delivery method that maximizes its potential—including the potential of attachment that is made easier through the direct contact of nursing and the hormones involved during this process. If you think about other mammals, I doubt any of those mothers are nursing their babies because they believe it is something they are meant to enjoy; instead, they do it because that is the means with which nature has provided them to feed their babies.

I've heard from numerous new mothers who feel guilty because they do not enjoy nursing their babies; they believe it is something they are meant to enjoy—a time of love and warm fuzzies. Sometimes women quit breastfeeding because they don't enjoy it and believe that they should. The "breast is best" campaign has set up the idea that if we are not breastfeeding, then by default we are doing something for our children that is less than the best— perhaps even damaging. But breastfeeding is not so much *best* as it is biologically *normal*. If we can return breastfeeding to its "normal" status, then we can overcome the concerns about whether we are giving or not giving our children the best, and instead, simply follow what is normal and biologically intended. Formula has its place; it is a lifesaving measure and necessary in many cases. But it is not normal. You are not doing something wrong if you do not love nursing your baby, and don't believe that every other mother loves it either.

Conversely, many articles, handbooks, and stories about breastfeeding refer to it as something to be endured. They provide "tips to survive the first days of breastfeeding". So many articles say breastfeeding can be difficult, and it can be painful. We set women up for failure by placing in their minds doubt and fear and struggle, instead of speaking of the natural means of approaching breastfeeding. By approaching it as normal and fighting against the view of breastfeeding as abnormal and the belief perpetuated by many baby supply companies that we need a plethora of "things" in order to breastfeed, we also reject the notion that we necessarily will have problems and difficulties. Too often, the difficulties and "failure" come from ignoring the natural process of breastfeeding and buying into the advertising and marketing plans of big business that would have us believe breastfeeding is challenging and hard and requires copious amounts of gadgets to get it right. The only gadgets and gizmos a mother truly needs are her breasts!

Our current societal view of breastfeeding seems to be quite superficial. There are many pleasantries and platitudes given, catchy phrases developed and disseminated, and outward encouragement extended to expectant and new mothers. But when looking on a deeper level, it doesn't take long to find the cracks in the support and discover its superficiality. Many hospitals do not have lactation support; health insurance rarely covers breast pumps that might be required in certain situations; employee lactation rooms have had to be legislated; milk banks struggle to secure adequate funding; nursing mothers are frequently being harassed and driven out of public places; and new mothers often have very little maternity leave available to them. It's no wonder many people question the value of breast milk when confronted with the reality of breastfeeding in our society.

When you consider the support given to artificial baby milk, or formula, the true lack of support for breastfeeding becomes clearly focused. Very few new mothers make it through pregnancy without receiving a sample of formula from a formula company; baby bottles are the go-to symbol used on baby related items such as cards, wrapping paper, advertising, and various types of literature (the Canadian government recently found it appropriate to use a baby bottle on the cover of a passport application); advertising for infant formula is ever-present in magazines, on television, and even in doctors' offices and hospitals in the form of freebies left behind by formula reps (check the tape measures used to check a baby's growth, for example). We are constantly being advertised to, being told that baby formula is normal, easy to use, and are often told that formula is "just like breast milk" or closest to breast milk. The power of multinational corporations is difficult to fight against. Breastfeeding is biologically normal and natural, but it doesn't have a marketing budget.

Those people who work tirelessly to promote breastfeeding and assist new mothers to breastfeed are often seen as being overzealous and pushy. New mothers will often complain that they were made to feel guilty or were judged for their decision not to breastfeed. New mothers who have difficulty breastfeeding sometimes say that the support they received was only support for breastfeeding and when they wanted to look at alternatives, they were made to feel that they were not doing what was best for their baby. As someone who exclusively pumped and wrote a book about exclusively pumping, I know all too well that options and alternatives to breastfeeding are rarely shared with new mothers who are struggling to breast-feed. Many women contact me saying that they had to "discover" the option of exclusively pumping on their own and that lactation support workers did not mention it as an alternative to them when they were going through breastfeeding difficulties.

At the other extreme are people who encourage formula feeding. Aside from formula manufacturers that obviously have financial motives to encourage the use of their products—and they certainly do encourage us to use them—there are people who are not convinced of breast milk's superiority and who will actively encourage new mothers to feed formula. This kind of pressure usually comes from family or friends. It can be based on the experience of the people encouraging formula feeding; if they fed their babies formula, they may feel that is the best choice for everyone. It can be based on inaccurate information; some people believe the hype of advertising campaigns that raise formula to the same level as breast milk. And sometimes it is based on body image, perceptions, and social mores; breasts are sexual objects, should not be bared in public, and a baby nursing is seen as disgusting or inappropriate.

How did our society come to this? And yet more importantly, how is a new mother to navigate these conflicting pressures and attitudes?

Consider Your Experience
I can honestly say that growing up in the 70s and 80s I never saw a mother nursing her baby. I was once in a house where a baby was breastfeeding, but that mother took the baby to the bedroom

to nurse. Baby bottles were how babies were fed, according to popular culture. Every baby doll that came into my house, or I saw in the stores, had a bottle accompanying it—after all, the baby had to eat, right? I learned all about sex in health class, including where babies come from, but I do not recall any mention of how babies are fed once they are born. Babies, again according to the popular culture of my childhood, were quiet, slept all the time, cooed and smiled, but only cried when hungry (which was easy enough to resolve with a bottle), played quietly on a blanket, and otherwise required little attention. How similar is this to the image of breastfeeding and babies that you grew up with? How similar is it to the image perpetuated today?

Today, formula manufacturers have overwhelmed the media. Formula is advertised in magazines, on television, in hospitals, through cross-promotion campaigns (think of companies that partner with formula manufacturers, sharing or selling mailing lists, or offering contests), and online. Some formula companies go so far as to offer breastfeeding advice—certainly no reason why they wouldn't want breastfeeding moms to be successful, right?

Consider your own experiences and the messages you have received about breastfeeding. Was it portrayed as something to be valued, encouraged, and supported, or something that was on the periphery, disdained, or old-fashioned? How much did you understand about newborns going into the experience of motherhood? Was it based on the knowledge of normal, biological behaviour? Or was it built from the perception of bottle-feeding being the normal method of infant nutrition? How can we expect mothers to be successful breastfeeding when our society has distanced itself from breastfeeding and instead transmits an understanding of bottle-feeding as the norm?

What, in fact, makes a new mother more likely to be successful at breastfeeding: whether she was breastfed, saw breastfeeding as a child, has family nearby, or lives in a big city? What about number of years married, years of education, country of citizenship, number of magazines or types of magazines read? Did she have an unmedicated birth or use a midwife? Does she have a certain yearly income level? Or is it some other intangible? Ultimately, does any of that matter? Many of these elements cannot be changed by an individual, and yet women that fall into all of these categories want to breastfeed, have difficulty breastfeeding, and need support to breastfeed. What matters far more than any of these elements is the simple way we as individuals, and we as a society, view breastfeeding.

Given that the nurturing and nourishment of our children is arguably the most important role we will have in our lives, we owe it to our children and ourselves to truly understand the duelling elements that impact the decisions we make about how to raise and care for our children. Our decision to breastfeed, and our ability to breastfeed, are two of the most interfered-with aspects of childrearing, and we as parents are for the most part unaware of this reality.[3]

Society's Views and Mothers' Choices

Breastfeeding is indeed an emotionally charged issue. The method by which you nourish your baby somehow becomes a topic of social importance. From the person sitting in the doctor's waiting room, to a mother you meet in the playground, to an older couple you pass in the grocery store, "Are you breastfeeding?" becomes a reasonable question for anyone to ask. Women who are breastfeeding may be judged by friends who do not understand why they can't attend a girls' night out at which children are not welcome. Just as your pregnant belly seemed to be publicly owned, so too is your feeding choice a social concern. Everyone seems to have an experience or opinion about breastfeeding.

And of course, there's the opposite experience: women who are formula feeding and who have to answer countless questions as to why they are not breastfeeding. If you are a mother who fully intended to breastfeed and for whom it did not work out, these questions are often painful and bring to the surface many emotions that you struggle to deal with. Put breast milk in a bottle, and the conversations often get much more complicated! And really, why does anyone feel the need to ask? Because breastfeeding—feeding in general—is such an emotional act.

In between the breastfeeding and formula feeding advocates are those who believe that breastfeeding is "best" for a baby but feel that it isn't always possible, doesn't always work out, and isn't the right choice for some women. A tour through internet discussion boards results in no shortage of comments from those sitting in the middle. Experienced mothers—often who had their own difficulties breastfeeding and more often than not did not have a successful, long-term breastfeeding experience—will tell a new mom who is having difficulties breastfeeding a number of things:

- Breastfeeding really isn't natural. You need to learn how to do it.
- Breastfeeding isn't as easy as you would think it should be.
- It can really hurt.
- It's really okay if you don't breastfeed.
- You've done your best.
- A lot of moms can't do it.
- A healthy baby is most important.
- A happy mommy equals a happy baby.
- Do what's best for you, and your baby.

On the surface, this all sounds great, but what does it all really mean? Is this what you really want to hear when you are going through a difficult experience? Is this truly helpful? If you were in the middle of an expedition to the top of Mount Everest would you want your companions encouraging you on by saying, "It's a big mountain. A lot of climbers never make it. It's okay if you quit now. You've done your best."? I really don't think so. Personally speaking, what would motivate me up that mountain is someone saying, "You can do it. You are strong and powerful. You've trained for this. Sure it's hard now, but you'll regret it if you don't push on." —and then I hope they'd pick up a bag, help me carry the burden, and climb with me to the top.

Our society is overcome with the fear of placing guilt on someone else—or adding to the guilt already felt—but in reality, only you can cause yourself to feel guilty. Guilt comes entirely from the knowledge that you have not done something you should have done, or the converse. Perhaps these helpful people in the middle of the breastfeeding-formula spectrum are trying to assuage the guilt still left over from their own experiences. Maybe this is even how you feel right now: guilt over your past experience, sadness and regret over the expectations lost, and resigned to believe that breastfeeding is truly a difficult, painful, challenging undertaking that often doesn't work out the way we hope. But this perspective is fuelled by our society's hang-ups, misinformation, and the market-driven economy. The best thing we as women can do to achieve normal breastfeeding is to be aware of those things that interfere with this desired outcome. Yet, while it is important to be aware, you can't always do it alone. For that reason you need to develop your support system.

Support Systems
One vital component of successful breastfeeding is the presence of a support system. Your support system may be very different

from mine, but the role is the same: to provide you with what you need to establish and maintain a long-term nursing relationship with your baby. There are many potential members of a support system including your spouse, your parents, your friends, your larger community, the health care system (doctors, nurses, lactation consultants, public health nurses), the society at large, and big business (formula and pump manufacturers, for example). Be aware that every person or organization you choose to include in your support system has the potential to either support or hinder your breastfeeding efforts — whether they are aware of it or not. It is for this reason that you need to choose carefully; consider each supporter's background, bias, and knowledge; and assess your ability to work with them, communicate with them, and accept help (and sometimes criticism) from them. If not chosen carefully, you might find that you include members into your circle of support who, through their own misinformation, either actively or passively encourage you to give up.

Consider the support system you had for your first breast-feeding experience. Consider their role honestly. Who in that support system encouraged you up the mountain and who told you it was okay to climb only half-way? Moving towards a new breastfeeding opportunity, it is crucial that you reflect on your support system, recognize what you need from your support system, and then put that support system in place *now*, before your baby is born, before you lose your ability to think rationally, and before you become overwhelmed with post-partum hormones and emotions. Begin now to make choices to surround yourself with positive supports. This includes the books and magazines you are reading, the doctor or midwife you choose, the companies to which you choose to give your money and with whom you share your contact information, and the visiting policies you put in place for friends and family during the immediate post-partum period.

And it is okay to limit access to you and your baby in the early days. In fact, this is a perfect job for daddy! Moms need protection from things that will cause stress, worry, or extra work, and that includes visits from people who are going to offer to feed your baby (even though they may know you are breast-feeding), ask what formula you are using, or suggest you simply bottle-feed since that's what they did and their children turned out "just fine".

Limiting access is also necessary for the incursions of big business into your home. Make it a standing policy to refuse to accept any free samples or gifts of formula. Ensure anyone throwing you a shower, or giving you gifts, knows that you intend to breastfeed and do not want any formula in your house. If you receive any formula or bottles as gifts, donate them to a food bank or throw them away. While all this might seem over the top, it's clear that having formula in the house when you are having difficulties breastfeeding creates a dangerous temptation to use it in a moment of emotion, exhaustion, and frustration. Ask yourself why formula companies are so willing to send full-sized cans of formula and large discount coupons to expectant and new mothers. They know that getting their product in your door enormously increases their chance of getting you as a customer. Your intention to breastfeed doesn't matter to them. You are a potential customer and they'll pursue you tirelessly to gain your money. Formula advertisements present bottle-feeding as a wonderful bonding moment between mom and baby: peaceful, quiet, easy. When you are in the midst of breastfeeding challenges, this serene image can be an enormous draw. It's a moment we all want to have with our child and many family members also have this desire.

The opportunity for a spouse or relative to feed the baby is a common reason why women want to be able to feed with a bottle: so they can share. Of course, biologically speaking, feeding is the role of the female of the species, but it is surely looked at as a bonding experience and this is why fathers and grandmothers want to be able to share in this experience. Recent research into oxytocin (a hormone connected to love and bonding) shows that levels of this hormone rise when people share a meal together. Perhaps bottle-feeding a baby causes a similar rise in oxytocin? Yet the fact remains that part of mothering, from a biological perspective, is the feeding of an infant. Mothers and babies biologically expect this relationship and interaction based on generations and generations of genetics and behaviours. When we choose to go against our biology, we choose to create within us an imbalance or lack of equilibrium. Is this perhaps the reason why mothers who chose not to breastfeed are so sensitive to others' comments and judgments surrounding the feeding of their child?

Of course it is vitally important that fathers and extended family bond with a new baby. But it is our society's error to believe that bonding happens best, or most easily, through feeding. Fathers fulfill an extremely important role in the life of an infant.[4] They are there, of course, to love and nourish a child, but they also can be the person other than the mother whom the baby learns to trust and enjoy. Diane Wiessinger, IBCLC, explains it best when she says to fathers, "Nursing and Mama are the center of a new baby's world. Nursing is his career, his hobby, his obsession. But his world keeps getting bigger, and the first person your baby will add to his world is you. You are The Safe Person Who Is Not Mama, and your very different style will gradually teach your baby that different can be nice, too." If we agree that breastfeeding is the biologically natural way of feeding, then we must also understand that fathers do not breastfeed. As Wiessinger points out, "For as long as there have been babies, there have been fathers. But no father in the history of the world ever nursed a baby."[5] If people feel so strongly about taking part in the feeding of a new baby, is there really any wonder why women have such emotional reactions to being unable to breastfeed? Support must come from everyone around us which includes well-meaning family and friends who feel that their ability to feed the baby is the only way they can bond with your child.

And support must also come from your doctor. Finding out after your baby's arrival that your doctor is not very knowledgeable about or supportive of breastfeeding can cause a great deal of grief. Imagine discovering that the one person you think should be supportive of breastfeeding really doesn't feel that strongly about it, is unable to give you accurate information, and perhaps even makes suggestions that will be detrimental to your efforts. This happens. The time to question your doctor about breastfeeding is not after your baby is born and difficulties arise, it is before your baby is born and while you still have options. While it would be wonderful to have all medical professionals well-versed in breastfeeding science and experienced working with breastfeeding moms, sadly, this isn't the case in our society. Many are well meaning and give the best information they have, but breastfeeding is not taught to any extent in medical school and unless a doctor is motivated to supplement their knowledge on their own, the support from your doctor may not be what you need or expect.

Aside from doctors, there are many others in the medical system who can strongly affect a new mother's breastfeeding success. Nurses in the hospital, both in the labour and delivery ward and the post-partum ward, lactation consultants, pharmacists, and health nurses all have a role to play in a mother and baby's breastfeeding relationship. I was mortified when my labour nurse stated immediately after my daughter was born — and I do mean immediately — that if she ever had a baby she would never breastfeed because it was simply too painful. This is not the kind of "support" a medical professional should be giving to new mothers, and yet it is not at all uncommon.

A website called *My OB Said What* contains numerous comments made to mothers during pregnancy, labour, and the postpartum period. Among the comments related to breastfeeding is one made to a mother one day after her baby was born and who reported breastfeeding was going well. The nurse declared, "Well things can change. Make sure you take these formula samples." Another young eighteen-year-old mother who intended to breastfeed was told by a nurse, "You are young and it hurts. You won't want to feel like a failure so do yourself a favor and give her the formula from the start." And it isn't only nurses that make unsupportive comments. An OB said to a mother who intended to breastfeed for an "extended" time, "Well, just be sure you don't breastfeed any longer than six months at most. You won't be happy with the shape of your breasts if you do." And as a final example, a lactation consultant stated to a tearful mother who was attempting to breastfeed her baby amid numerous complications, "There are women here who are *serious* about breastfeeding you know."[6] Recognizing that not everyone who *should* support breastfeeding does support it is an important step in moving forward from a devastating breastfeeding experience and figuring out how to make it work the second time. Medical professionals are just people, and while they should be there to support their patients, the fact is that we are all affected by the same outside influences.

Setting Us Up for Failure

So this is where we're at. We are biological creatures. We are mammals, which means we are intended to feed our infants breast milk. Our babies are also born with a host of innate reflexes and skills that allow them to seek out the breast, locate the nipple, latch on, and suckle to remove milk. And yet our society fails to recognize breasts for their intended use, choosing instead to focus on the sexual and aesthetic aspects of a woman's body. Society also markets and advertises infant formula to new mothers, fails to provide significant breastfeeding support, and creates birthing conditions that are detrimental to a successful mother/baby nursing relationship. In fact, given the conditions under which many babies are born, it's miraculous that we have as many breastfed babies as we do.

This connection between birthing practices and breastfeeding is particularly interesting. It is valuable to question the overall perception of birth and how the current attitude and understanding of birth affect our ability to breastfeed. As previously mentioned, c-section rates are soaring in North America and it is uncommon to hear a woman recount her birth story and not have it include some type of intervention, and more often multiple interventions. Women like to share the horrors of childbirth, but rarely do women hear about positive birth experiences; the ones that didn't require drugs, monitoring, or surgery (and sadly the same is true for breastfeeding stories). The positive stories are out there, but all too often they need to be searched out. They are not part of the common literature of first pregnancies.

Our society has come to accept that babies are born in a hospital; that childbirth is painful and pain management is required (or else you are looked at as a martyr or crazy person); that doctors always know what's best when it comes to birth; and that directly following birth babies must be assessed, monitored, weighed, injected, and tested in order to ensure their survival. We as women have been completely disconnected from our bodies and made to believe that pregnancy and childbirth are medical conditions. How does this general acceptance of pregnancy and birth then relate to breastfeeding? Is it possible that our beliefs about childbirth are affecting our ability to breastfeed?

When I became pregnant with my first child I asked my mother about her memories of pregnancy, childbirth, and breastfeeding. Even though I was thirty-one years old, I had never thought to ask her about these experiences and didn't even know if I had been breastfed. I was amazed and perplexed when she told me she remembered nothing about childbirth. It was shortly after that that I discovered women during that time period were frequently put into "twilight sleep" during labour and delivery. Doctors provided a mix of drugs that created an amnesiac effect but did not provide any significant pain management.[7]

New mothers would "wake up" with a baby in their arms and no memory of the events that led up to that moment. Is this what happened in my mother's case? Is it possible that twilight sleep was still in use in the early 1970s? And how would an experience such as this impact breastfeeding? To be so disconnected from your body's strength and ability during childbirth might also disconnect you from its strength and ability as it relates to breastfeeding.

One of the most difficult aspects of breastfeeding failure to overcome is the loss of faith we have in our bodies, our babies, and ourselves. It can be exceedingly difficult to let go of the "failure," determine the true causes, and accept that our bodies did not fail us, our babies did know what they were doing, and that we have the ability to make it work. But what happens when the false stories about our bodies' inability to live up to biological expectations are told to us during pregnancy, brought to fruition during childbirth due to interference from the medical system, and then continued into the post-natal period as we attempt to establish a breastfeeding relationship with our new child? Women are being told that their bodies do not work. This is simply untrue. What doesn't work is the current medical system—a system that would have a woman believe that she needs a c-section to birth her child or that she would never be able to manage labour without an epidural. Is it such a far reach to connect this same attitude to the failure of mothers to produce milk or to latch a baby?[8]

It would appear that we have failed at birthing with sky-rocketing rates of epidurals, c-sections, and other interventions that are presented to us as necessary and unavoidable. Are we also establishing a societal belief that as women we cannot do what we were designed to do? Does having a poor birthing experience cause us to see ourselves as more likely to "fail" at breastfeeding which then leads to the fruition of that belief? There are certainly physiological reasons why certain birth interventions make breastfeeding more challenging, but important too is the recognition of the psychological effects of birth interventions and the feeling of inability and failure that they create. Think back to your own pregnancy and subsequent breastfeeding attempt. What was your birthing experience like? Did it create a sense of trust and belief in your body and your body's ability to do what it was designed to do? Or did it instead create doubt and fear in you and chisel away at the faith you might have had in your body and the process?

In my own experience, my first pregnancy and delivery certainly did cause me to question my body's ability. It was my body's failure, its weakness and illness, that forced my son to be born at only thirty-one weeks gestation. I clearly remember thinking that my body had failed him, and for this reason, breastfeeding was that much more important to me. However, when breastfeeding proved unsuccessful, in my mind it was proven as fact that my body simply could not do what it was designed to do. It was only through extensive reading of what some might consider "alternative" pregnancy and childbirth books, working through my emotions relating to the lost breast-feeding relationship, and beginning to recognize what I was capable of and that I had done the best I could given my knowledge, support, and understanding at the time, that I was able to move into my second pregnancy with a renewed sense of ability and faith.

You May Need to Adjust Your Set

Our technologically connected world allows for significant opportunities to disseminate information and ideology about breastfeeding. Sometimes these messages are supportive and positive, but all too often they are based on the desired monetary gains of big business. These messages can be aimed at all age groups and show just how ingrained and accepted bottle-feeding has become in our society. In 1977, Buffy St. Marie appeared on *Sesame Street* breastfeeding her young son, Cody.[9] St. Marie's appearance on the show with her son was a wonderful normalization of breastfeeding and undoubtedly an eye-opener for a generation of children that may not have otherwise been exposed to breastfeeding. Mister Rogers even saw fit to have an episode on nursing. Today, however, breastfeeding is not as prevalent in children's programming.

My daughter loves Dora, but unfortunately even Dora, who has access to millions of young girls, normalizes bottle-feeding. In the episode called "Big Sister Dora," Dora's mother has twins and Dora arrives home to meet her new baby brother and sister and help bottle-feed one of them. I also remember my children watching an episode of *Zaboomafoo* that was all about baby animals. It discussed how baby animals were fed. But when it came time to discuss baby humans, there was a bottle in the baby's mouth and not a mention of breastfeeding. A great opportunity to share breastfeeding with children—missed.

Of course parents have the right to choose how they should care for their children; however, it is important to question the messages we have been exposed to throughout our lives and question truly to what extent our choices are our own. If we are not given the complete picture, or are given half-truths, or if we are targeted by advertising to such an extent that we, without even thinking, grab for one product over another without being able to verbalize why we are making the choice, then we truly are not free to make a choice; our choices are being made for us. If children are never exposed to breastfeeding, never taught that breastfeeding is a normal way to feed an infant, is that a choice that we expect them to make when they have children of their own?

Marketing also greatly influences our choices as parents. A significant percentage of the content of parenting magazines is advertising and often articles and information are simply thinly veiled advertisements. Even companies that one would think support breastfeeding, such as breast pump manufacturers, may be more interested in promoting their product and use messages to distance a new mom from the normal process of breastfeeding. Michelle, a mother who struggled with social pressures when attempting to establish a breastfeeding relationship with her son, clearly recognized the impact of marketing surrounding breastfeeding and breastfeeding support explaining, "The amount of advice and counselling one could get, the sheer numbers of contraptions one could invest in, the full gamut of the books that were available for sale came at me with a dizzying pace leaving me utterly bewildered." The commodification of breastfeeding, making it into a money-making venture, moves breastfeeding away from being a normal process and towards being a mechanical and medical process that requires effort and, most of all, purchases.

And distancing women from the normal process is exactly what many companies are doing. A recent marketing campaign by a large pump manufacturer had significant shelf space in a very popular American department store. The campaign suggested that everything needed in order to breastfeed was a breast pump, accessories, and self-care. Of course the shelves were filled with the company's products. What kind of message is this marketing really sending to mothers? Is there really anything that you need in order to breastfeed? Last time I checked, a breast pump was not a requirement. All I can see that you really need is a baby and breasts. Yet companies teach us that our bodies are not enough, that we need to spend money on gadgets and accessories, and that we are not enough on our own. Cynthia Good Mojab asserts that there is a lack of "knowledge, skill, and maturity" with regards to the task of mothering and that many women are completely unprepared for the experience of motherhood. She believes that "This in fact indicates a tragic failure of social systems—not a tragic failure of individual women." Referencing the plethora of gadgets and devices aimed at mothers and babies Good Mojab states: "According to the marketing, such conflicts between expectations and reality can only be solved with the purchase of a product: a tape of a mother's heart beat that plays any time baby stirs from sleep, artificial substitutes for human milk, more and more toys..."[10] As Good Mojab indicates, the impact of marketing and our society in general strongly affects how we view motherhood and our expectations for motherhood. While it may be impossible to avoid all these influences—and likely not even desired—being aware of them will help you to limit the impact.

As you move towards a second opportunity to breastfeed, consider the messages that you have been given with regards to your body and your abilities. Consider the birth process and how it may affect what happens following birth. Refuse to feel guilty about doing what your doctors told you was needed and proper, and doing what you knew was best at that point in time. Instead, recognize that you, as a woman, were created to birth your children and nourish them at your breast. Embrace the biological aspects of your being and refuse to accept the message too often suggesting that women are unable to birth their own children without a doctor and medical intervention. Your past experience is your past experience, but you do not need to be defined or confined by it. While your first experience may not have been what you wanted it to be, it does not predict or limit your next experience. There are no guarantees, but through thoughtful examination of your own knowledge, feelings, values and beliefs, societal influences, and support network, you can work towards a much more positive experience—an experience that will allow you to make decisions and base them on the knowledge and belief that you *were* intended to breastfeed, and you *can* determine what it means to be successful.

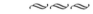

Caroline's Story

Before getting pregnant I would definitely have described myself as pro-breastfeeding. I had strong feelings and even a bit of attitude about those who chose not to breastfeed. I had grown up listening to stories about how my mother breastfed me until thirteen months of age—the day I started unbuttoning her blouse on the Toronto streetcar. I always based my expectations on her experiences, and just assumed I would nurse the same amount.

When I was in my late twenties, I married and experienced fertility challenges. It was startling because my mom was pregnant first-try with me, so I had been very vigilant with birth control and condoms. After a few years, I switched family doctors and with the first physical examination discovered I had two inverted nipples. I didn't even know what they were! I Googled "inverted nipples" and discovered they might make breastfeeding more challenging, but had no idea what that could mean. I didn't give it another thought.

Then, as my friends started having babies, one in particular shared with me that breastfeeding had been a big learning curve—that the blissful descriptions we read about in books, the immediate latch in the delivery room, are not the norm. I listened more carefully to the section on breastfeeding during the pre-natal classes, but it still seemed very foreign. I was sure my body would "just know" what to do. I watched my previously very timid friend "whip out her boob" at my baby shower, and later listened to family and friends aghast at her "display". This just made me more resolved to be a poster girl for breastfeeding.

I am now the mother of four children: Anthony (soon 6), Jack (soon 4), and 6 month-old twins, Michael and Emma. And with these four children, I have gained a wealth of breastfeeding experience. When Anthony was born, after an induction for intrauterine growth restriction, I brought him to my breast. There was nothing to latch on to, so nothing happened. No opening of the skies and lady Madonna moment. So the nurse in the delivery room and my mother tried to "tickle" my nipple to make it erect. Nothing. The nurse then brought a syringe with one open end, placed it on my nipple, and drew suction. My toes curled! Still nothing. Now there was a lady waiting to get to the delivery room, and I was refusing to be moved back to my room until my baby had latched.

Back in my room, the nurse looked aghast at the syringe con-traption, explained I might damage my nipple tissues, and suggested I needed to use a pump…"Oh, but none are available at the moment." So I waited. And then pumped and tried and...you get the picture. Each nurse that came into my room contradicted the one before her.

So after a few days, it was time to go home. Instead of renting, my parents had bought me an Ameda pump. I "nursed" Anthony every few hours, and pumped for twenty minutes after that, but still no sign of milk. That night, he started crying. And then the milk came in. I awoke in a puddle—and pumped 12 oz.!

That afternoon, we had our home visit from the public health nurse. She came to the house, weighed him, and then expressed concern that he was completely dehydrated! His diaper was full of crystals. All these days of nursing, and he wasn't getting anything! So she pulled out a Monojet syringe and taught my hubbie and me to slide it along our fingers and feed him the pumped milk. She also explained that there was a lactation consultant available the next day at the health unit.

The lactation consultant was great! She ushered us in and spent thirty minutes with us. She was delighted that I had the "Breast Buddy" nursing pillow, and recommended I go to the pharmacy and buy breast shields.

So began my six months of nursing with the shield, then pumping for twenty minutes, then feeding some expressed milk, and then freezing the rest. I was always concerned that my son wasn't getting enough. He never became a plump, healthy looking baby. He is still a small guy at six.

I would go to mother's circle and try to nurse with everyone. As the time wore on, Anthony got fussier and fussier. No matter my intent to nurse wherever and however, my body was too tense in public. I remember pulling out a bottle of expressed milk at my old worksite and was quite offended when someone thought it was formula (instead of the liquid gold).

Anthony was born in June, and by December I was down to only seeing 0.5 oz. at a pumping. I tried days of intensive pumping every two hours, and there was no effect on my supply. A friend explained that it was because my breast was not receiving any skin-to-skin contact. So I decided to abandon it altogether, and switch to formula. A nightmare of trying Good Start…and then a rash…and then trying soy-based…and still more rashes.

Halfway through my second pregnancy, I went into a tailspin. I suffered from severe depression and needed medication. I was given the options for post-delivery. I was at a 70% risk of severe post-partum depression. I could nurse, or take the meds. I reluctantly opted for the meds, and feel like I suffered just as much by feeling like a failure as a mother. Jack was a healthy, happy boy and grew rapidly. I didn't go to any groups because I didn't feel I belonged.

I still keep the mantra in my head that I chose to be a mother, instead of a food source, to him and his brother.

Maybe the second experience is why I felt so strongly that I wasn't finished having children. I had always talked about having four kids if we won a lottery. But when my husband and I had married, he wanted one and we agreed to stop at two.

My last pregnancy, my beautiful twins, feels like a partial recovery—a chance to "do it all right". Instead of meds, I opted to reduce and stop stressors. I changed jobs in advance, and continued to seek out more therapy and treatments. I have ended up being really casual about my breastfeeding with the twins. Less obsessed, but not the total success I would have hoped for. I am not ready to nurse exclusively (part of my no-meds plan requires more sleep). I tell people I nurse, and lie to the doctor about the amounts. I don't want it to end, but I am now pumping about twenty drops at a time. At least I was able to stop using the shields sometimes because the suction from the breast pump released the tension inverting my nipples and my babies could latch without this aid.

So much of how I view myself as a mother is tied to nursing. It doesn't make any sense. My husband doesn't understand why I keep putting this stress on myself, especially when there is so much at risk for my mood. It's a fine balancing act, and one I feel I am losing. Feeling as though I had no part in the decision not to nurse my second son, Jack, made me adamant about wanting the nursing experience again. But as soon as the twins cry, I wonder if they are getting enough, and quickly stuff in a bottle of formula.

My feelings about breastfeeding have dramatically changed. Ironically I would never sign up to be a breastfeeding buddy at the health unit because I don't feel I could advocate enough in favour of breastfeeding. I feel jaded about breastfeeding. Anthony had eczema, ear infections, and rashes. These weren't supposed to happen to a breastfed baby. Jack, who never had breast milk, has had none of these problems.

I feel huge guilt about not solely breastfeeding the twins and Jack. I let myself off the hook around others with lots of justifications, but in my own head they are just excuses. Using formula feels like a cop-out. I envy my friends who have breastfed (and tandem nursed) their children until four or five years of age. Then when they suffer through the pangs of trying to wean I secretly think…well that's what you get. It's awful of me!

I'm still in it. Today I held the twins, crying and trying to stuff their faces with a boob. I have the bottle beside me, but I won't give it until they have had a few sucks. They seem so miserable. They finally give in and spend ten to twenty seconds of exhausted suckling. Then they resume the crying. I thought about going to rent the Medela again at Shoppers, then doing an intensive week of pumping to get my supply up, or making an appointment with my doctor to get the milk-making medicine. I'm not ready for this to be over. There will be no more babies, and no more nursing. I remember how sad I was when I couldn't nurse Jack and I'm not ready to face that again.

The Unknown "Why"

"I was told by one nurse that my positioning was fine and that pain was normal. Another nurse told me I should have no pain and to alter my positioning. Nothing helped."

Flora, mother of one

So just what is breastfeeding "failure"? What does it mean? And who determines whether or not a mother is successful? Early weaning, early supplementation, exclusively pumping, not attempting to breastfeed at all...are all these considered to be breastfeeding failure? There are wide-ranging reasons for breastfeeding challenges. Ultimately, breastfeeding failure has more to do with your own perspective on the subject—your own expectations and intentions—than with a certain length of time you breastfed or the exclusivity of breastfeeding. We, as new mothers, often allow others to judge our ability as mothers. We read magazines and watch television shows that suggest what it means to be a good mother. Images are constantly presented to us in society that show new mothers dressed well, out and about, well rested, make-up on, with not a care in the world. Those of us who are mothers also know that this image is far from reality.

While we may work hard to present an image of having it all together, most new moms I know feel they're a long way from matching up to this media image. So when it comes to breastfeeding, are we also letting others determine our success or tell us what success looks like? Are we trying to reach unattainable goals? Do we understand what is normal when it comes to breastfeeding and do we create realistic goals, determining our own success? Are we being unfair to ourselves by allowing others to judge whether we are breastfeeding *successfully* or whether we are a breastfeeding *failure*? Having a clear understanding of what is normal for breastfeeding, how to follow the natural course of breastfeeding in order to increase the chances of success, and how to set your own goals for determining success can all help mothers to become successful at breastfeeding and to leave the idea of breastfeeding failure in the past.

Real Reasons for Breastfeeding "Failure"

There are three main reasons for breastfeeding difficulties in our modern world: 1.) a lack of knowledge, 2.) a lack of support, and 3.) pressures from society. Breastfeeding difficulties and subsequent early weaning might appear to have a root cause of a low milk supply, pain that was insurmountable, a baby's preference for a bottle nipple, or the impact of an underlying medical condition, but in truth lack of success almost always relates back to one of these three causes coupled with an unwavering standard of what defines "successful breastfeeding".

As a first time mother with a thirty-one week preemie, I certainly faced all of the above challenges. And perhaps using my own experience is the best way to explain how these three elements over-ride all other aspects of breastfeeding failure. Someone else looking at my experience may suggest my lack of success was a result of exhaustion, a lack of dedication, the impact of my son's severe reflux, my pain from thrush, my separation from my son for the first eighteen hours of his life and continued separation while he was in the NICU, or poor support once he was released from the hospital. The list of reasons could go on and on. None of these judgements would be entirely accurate, and some would certainly not be fair. Ultimately, it's your own judgement that's important—not the judgement of those around you. And in reality, I think all breastfeeding challenges come down to a combination of these three elements: a lack of knowledge, a lack of support, and the impact of societal pressures.

About a week before my son was born I had visited my local library and borrowed a number of books on breastfeeding. This was seven months into my pregnancy. I had already completed my prenatal course at the local hospital; and honestly I can't remember any breastfeeding instruction as part of that course. If it was there, it was definitely a cursory level of information. My family doctor had never mentioned breastfeeding during prenatal visits. I didn't know anyone who had breastfed; I was not breastfed as a baby; and I had never even seen a baby being breastfed. Unfortunately, I don't think this is all that uncommon for women of my generation.

I am an information junkie by nature and love the opportunity to learn about a new topic, especially if that topic is one that is affecting me directly. So I pored over books about pregnancy and childbirth—and yet breastfeeding was not even on my radar. I knew I wanted to breastfeed, but never thought of needing to educate myself about it. Funny. Childbirth will happen regardless of what we do or don't do, know or don't know. That baby will come out! But while breastfeeding is something that is crucial to the development of our babies, a relationship that can continue for a couple of years or longer, and an integral part of the mother-baby life once our babies are born, I didn't consider it important, or perhaps more accurately didn't consider it necessary, to put more time into learning about breastfeeding than I did childbirth. This is part one of my lack of information.

Once my son was born, information on breastfeeding was intermittent, and the type of support received was not always what I needed. The NICU my son was in had three full-time lactation consultants. Access to help was not a problem. However, no breastfeeding instruction was ever given to me directly. No one explained the process of lactation or how supply is controlled. No one ever thought to question how I was feeling about the situation in which I found myself.

The first time I attempted to breastfeed my son, an overzealous nurse physically, and forcefully, handled my son and my breast leaving me with a very negative feeling about the experience. The second time I attempted to breastfeed, a nurse suggested I use a nipple shield and the lactation consultant, upon entering the room, stated, "So I hear you want to use a nipple shield." I had no idea what a nipple shield was let alone whether I wanted to use one. I just wanted it to work out and for my son to come home. No mention of the possible impact of a nipple shield was ever mentioned, simply the warning was given to ensure I continued pumping while using it because my supply could drop otherwise.

When I questioned why my son was continually, and increasingly, spitting up, no one ever mentioned that a high number of preemies develop gastrointestinal reflux disorder (GERD) and often require medication. When I asked why he was screaming and thrashing, the advice was to swaddle him tightly to control his hands. Again, no mention of the possibility of GERD. One of the lactation consultants, without any discussion with me, pointedly stated that she wanted my baby fully breastfeeding before he went home. This was after almost two weeks in a mother/baby unit with me stuck in an eight-by-ten foot room twenty-four hours a day with no end in sight. While my son was growing well, breastfeeding was becoming more and more difficult due to his screaming and thrashing during and after feedings. And the final piece of advice given in the hospital was from a well-meaning nurse who told me that if it were her, she would just use a bottle in order to get out of the hospital because babies in the hospital often contract other diseases. Talk about a way to scare a new mother into bottle-feeding!

Outside of the hospital, the poor information and lack of support continued. The lactation support from the hospital was not available on an outpatient basis, so I needed to find a new support system. Of course this hadn't been arranged prior to having my son, so I, in a state of exhaustion, stress, and shell shocked from my own illness (preeclampsia) and the experience of having a thirty-one week preemie, had to forge a new relationship in order to find information and support. A local nurse from the health unit made a home visit, and I was able to see her at a local well-baby drop-in clinic. Yet though I continued to voice my concerns about my son's difficulties breastfeeding, it did not seem that they were heeded, and I was told everything seemed fine. But everything wasn't fine. I was eventually told that it was okay to switch to formula if that is what I wanted. I'd tried my best and it was okay to stop. This was most definitely *not* what I wanted, but I couldn't get anyone to listen to me or stop long enough to truly understand my concerns.

My own experiences highlight not a failure on my part, but a lack of information. It wasn't my failure to properly recognize or manage my son's reflux that caused our problems; nor was it the separation that was forced upon us given the circumstances surrounding his birth. No, instead the real culprit here was the lack of information I had about how to manage breastfeeding in the face of these challenges.

Lack of Knowledge

While it should be an easy problem to resolve, the lack of information about breastfeeding for new mothers is shocking and is a contributing factor to dismal breastfeeding rates.[1] In an age of information, where anything you wish to know can be found at your fingertips on the internet, there is also a deluge of misinformation, half-truths, and out-and-out lies available. New mothers are not immune to this. While information may be available, it is extremely difficult to wade through the mountains of information present in books and from online sources and recognize what is accurate and valuable—and what is not. Many corporate interests involve themselves in the information game, providing marketing in the guise of information. It's no wonder breastfeeding mothers have a hard time finding reliable information when they desperately need it.

You'd hope that information would be easier to find in hospitals and from doctors, but this is often not the case. While some doctors are very breastfeeding friendly, there is a noticeable lack of information given to students in medical schools. Dr. Michelle Gibson, C.C.F.D., explains that "out of four years of medical school there may be only one lecture on breastfeeding."[2] Doctors who go on to a residency in family medicine will have the opportunity for additional training and to follow several women from pregnancy through the early post-partum period, but there is no guarantee of any in-depth breastfeeding training during this time. Often the primary experience a doctor has with regards to breastfeeding is with his or her own child; and information that arises from personal experience can obviously be biased. It's important to remember and acknowledge that medical professionals are part of the same society that we are part of and their position does not remove them from the influences of society and marketing.

It can be challenging to discern whether a doctor's advice is being given from a medical, evidence-based perspective or from a personal perspective, but it would be unfair to think that doctors should be able to always separate the two. Dr. Gibson explains that while lactation and breastfeeding education for doctors is improving, there is a hidden curriculum at play:

what's valued compared to what is taught. Also, doctors tend to see the worst of the worst in terms of breastfeeding related problems and their clear understanding of just how sick a baby can get when she is not breastfeeding well can lead doctors to sometimes encourage options such as supplementation.

Ultimately, medical doctors work within a health system that has limitations and weaknesses. Dr. Gibson laments, "Even the best physicians who are passionate about breastfeeding and breast milk are hamstrung by the lack of support."[3] Doctors tend to be overworked, have limited time, and have a limited number of community resources to which they can refer their patients. The lack of support that women face when breastfeeding is felt also by our doctors.

The challenges of a system lacking in support is also felt by Sandy Stevenson, an IBCLC working in Ontario, Canada. She explains

> I think a big part of the problem with professional breastfeeding support is fragmentation—each mother sees many, many health care providers. Women see one caregiver after another as they move along the continuum of their birth and breastfeeding experience (family physician, office staff, prenatal educator, midwife, obstetrician, (many) hospital nurses, paediatrician, (several) public health nurses, nurse practitioner, lactation consultant). Then to compound the problem, much of the advice breastfeeding women get from these many sources is outdated and wrong. As the IBCLC, I am at the end of the long line of health care providers, and I usually have to help the mother to sort through all the conflicting, inaccurate advice she has received. No wonder women are confused and don't know whom to trust! No wonder they have breastfeeding problems! The least we should do (as health care providers in a

fragmented system) is to ensure that we are all giving the best evidence-based information. Although much work is going on to meet this goal (like the Baby-Friendly Initiative), we still have a long way to go to provide great professional support to breastfeeding women everywhere.[4]

Judith Gutowski, an IBCLC working in the United States, sees the same issues when trying to provide new mothers with accurate information. She shares

Previously, I worked in private practice where the mothers didn't find me until the problems had been ongoing for two or more weeks. By that time milk supplies that could have been normal are low due to poor breast stimulation and babies have no energy due to weight loss and their feeding skills have declined due to supplementing, and so on. The longer a breastfeeding problem is not recognized and managed the harder it is to normalize.[5]

These two accounts from IBCLCs show how challenging the system is to navigate not only for new mothers, but also for the professionals working within the system. Mothers may reach out for help and information, but all too often they do not know who to listen to, who to believe. Within the hospital setting, Gutowski asserts

...it is not the norm for the hospitals in the U.S. to have adequate breastfeeding support available for their patients...For the sake of the bottom line, hospitals will often cut lactation care which is seen as a non-necessity...Due to these reasons, many mothers have not received even good basic breastfeeding support and information as part of maternity care. They are usually at home before the milk comes in and that is when the problems become apparent.[6]

New mothers need information and need to be able to trust the information they are getting. Currently, the system seems to be making this difficult and mothers are left trying to navigate a system that does not give breastfeeding education and support the appropriate emphasis and priority it deserves.

We are raised in our society to view doctors as people who have authority and power and this can lead us to accept their recommendations and direction without question. If you haven't already spoken to your doctor about breastfeeding, make a point of doing so. Labour and delivery, and the early post-partum period, are times when as new mothers we may feel particularly vulnerable and may not be as confident and outspoken as during other times of our lives. Having a frank discussion with your doctor before your new baby is born will help you to understand your doctor's attitudes and knowledge and forge a partnership based on a common goal.

While a discussion with your doctor is a great place to start, the truth of the matter is that many new moms get bad information and advice. This is the truth of our situation as new mothers. We look to those who should know and we trust the information we are given. When that advice is bad advice, it negatively affects the outcome and sometimes this means we are not successful in our efforts to breastfeed. As Maya Angelou says, "When you know better, you do better." A mother can't be faulted for doing what she was told was best, but we as a society *are* responsible for failing mothers and babies. Better information is needed. Mothers need access to good information. Mothers need to know that the information they receive is not merely a marketing ploy and that it is not biased by someone's personal experience or viewpoint.

It is important to point out that responsibility for the information received from doctors and lactation consultants lands on the mother as well as the professional being consulted. Sandy Stevenson, IBCLC, relates that "What is heard by the mother is not always what was said. In the heat of hormones, pain and fatigue, even accurate, well-meant advice might not be heard the way it was intended or said."[7] It's completely understandable why a new mother may not correctly hear what a doctor or lactation consultant is saying, but it is important to do everything possible to ensure the information is received accurately. Having the doctor or lactation consultant write down their instructions, for example, can help in clarifying instructions and aiding the foggy memory of the post-partum period. It is also highly recommended that you always take someone else with you when you visit the doctor or lactation consultant. This person can help you to both clarify and remember what was said.

Aside from doctors, a mother might also seek assistance from a lactation consultant. Unfortunately, the term "lactation consultant" is quite poorly defined and anyone can call themselves a lactation consultant. I often have women complain about the lack of information or the inaccurate information they received from a lactation consultant, but there is no guarantee that the person they saw was a board certified lactation consultant (IBCLC). To ensure you are receiving the best information possible, ask about the credentials of the person giving you advice and assistance.

There are numerous situations in which new moms need to have accurate and timely information in order to make decisions on how to manage their breastfeeding relationship. The following are some of those situations. Perhaps you will have had personal experience with some of them. As you read through the following information, consider your own experience. Do any of these seem familiar? Now from the distance of time, can you see your experience a bit more clearly and, placing blame aside, analyse it critically? The first step in changing your experience, is under-standing it.

Failure to Latch

One common reason given for breastfeeding failure is the inability of a newborn to latch. Some babies do not seem to latch at all, and some may latch but do so inconsistently or ineffec-tively. When faced with this reality, a mother has several options, and the opportunity for breastfeeding, once the situation improves, depends largely on the type of information the mother has access to and the quality of support she has around her.

Many problems with a baby's latch can often be overcome, but timely access to accurate information is important. A baby that isn't latching or transferring sufficient quantities of milk presents a large challenge to breastfeeding, but not having the information you need to make good choices in order to handle these types of problems often leads to devastating results. Over the years, I've heard from many women whose babies didn't latch immediately after birth and breastfeeding initiation was delayed. Too often in these cases women were not told that they should begin pumping to initiate supply and avoid problems down the road. A baby who is having trouble with latching and milk transfer is going to have a much more difficult time if there is no milk to be had. Yet information about early stimulation and pumping if a baby is not latching is not consistently given to women. I have grieved with far too many women who have discovered too late that the information and support they needed in those early days of breastfeeding was not given to them.

Mothers whose babies are not latching, or not latching well, often fall into the practice of bottle-feeding to either supplement what the baby is receiving at the breast, or in place of breastfeed-ing. Without clear and accurate information on how to initiate and protect her milk supply, and information, support and follow-up to assist her to transition baby to the breast, bottle-feeding often becomes the primary method of feeding in very short order. It may not be a conscious choice, and many mothers feel that they do not receive support for other options.

One such option is exclusively pumping. Too often women feel if breastfeeding doesn't work out that formula feeding is the only other option, but this simply isn't true. The World Health Organization (WHO) recognizes formula feeding as the fourth option for infant nutrition coming after a mother's expressed milk and donor milk, with direct breastfeeding of course being the first choice.[8] Many women who end up exclusively pumping do so thinking they are all alone in their venture. But they are not! Exclusively pumping is a long-term alternative to formula feeding and protects a mother's milk supply providing the option to return to breastfeeding should the problems be resolved.[9] Exclusively pumping certainly isn't the easiest choice, but it is another option when breastfeeding is not going well .

Pain

Pain associated with breastfeeding can be excruciating. Finding the motivation to face toe-curling pain every couple of hours in order to continue breastfeeding can be enormously difficult. Couple this pain with a lack of sleep, lack of information, lack of support, and the hormonal roller coaster of the post-partum period, and pain can become a legitimate reason for early weaning. Yet breastfeeding really shouldn't be painful. Think about it. Does it make sense that the biological means of feeding our babies should be something that is painful? Does it make sense, evolutionarily speaking, to have the means of nutrition for infants be something that mothers have an aversion to? I don't think so. And yet it is a fact that many new breastfeeding mothers experience pain when breastfeeding. This pain often is limited to the first couple of weeks and then resolves, at least to a manageable level, but when in the midst of the battle, avoiding the cause of the pain can make a lot more sense to us than persevering. Without accurate information and support, there often appears to be no end in sight and moms often feel the need to turn to a method of self-preservation. It's kind of like the old joke about the man who goes to his doctor and says that his hand hurts when he hits it, so his doctor tells him to stop hitting it.

Failure to Thrive

It can be terrifying to have a baby diagnosed as "failure to thrive". No mother wants to be told her baby is not growing as he should—especially when breastfeeding. There are many reasons a baby might be labelled as failure to thrive: medical issues, severe reflux, inefficient latch, metabolic issues. A low milk supply or inefficient milk transfer can cause slow growth. Often, formula supplementation is used to help boost a baby's intake, and with this intervention comes a whole host of risks to continued breastfeeding. But what is a mother to do? Your doctor tells you your baby is not thriving. You may internalize the issue feeling as though you are at fault for your baby's slow growth. You may not have access to any lactation support. Formula and a bottle seem like a solution to the problem. Even though it is not what you want, and certainly not what you planned, you need to feed your baby, and so baby gets fed formula, mother's milk supply diminishes, and eventually complete weaning has taken place.

Milk Supply Concerns

Our society values the ability to measure and quantify every-thing. And yet as a new breastfeeding mother, we are unable to measure the amount of milk our babies are taking. Combine this with a lack of information about normal infant feeding and behaviour, and the not-so-subtle pressure from formula companies to use their products, and you have created the perfect situation for a new mom to question her abilities and her body. A low milk supply, whether it is a true low supply or a perceived low supply, is one of the most common reasons new mothers give for supplementing and early weaning. As mothers we want to care for our babies; it is wired into us. Part of the care we give is the nourishment we provide. But what happens when we are unable to provide enough nourishment for our babies? The emotional impact of this can be devastating.

A true low milk supply is often caused by poor breastfeeding management and early supplementation with formula. However, there are physiological reasons why new mothers may have a low supply of milk (e.g. PCOS, diabetes, hypoplastic breasts). Regardless of the reasons or realities, the fear of not having enough milk for your baby can be very strong and create great anxiety. Our world is one that quantifies everything. Not being able to quantify the amount of milk your baby is receiving but continuing to breastfeed anyway can be a leap of faith in our number-obsessed world.

From my own experience, I can easily relate to this aspect of breastfeeding failure. Although I did produce enough milk for both of my children, with my attempts to breastfeed my son, the concern about how much he was getting became a huge obsession. With my son, who was born at thirty-one weeks and spent five weeks in the NICU after his birth, breastfeeding was difficult. I desperately wanted to breastfeed, and was using a breast pump to initiate and maintain my milk supply in the hopes that my son would be able to transition to breastfeeding once he got stronger, but the message I heard from the hospital was one of numbers: volumes, weight, number of hours between feedings. An article I wrote about my battle with the numbers is included at the end of the chapter.

Separation

Separation of a mother and baby is heartbreaking regardless of the reasons for it. Both mothers and babies can suffer from the absence of the other. When separated, a baby still must be fed and a mother, if she wishes to breastfeed, must express her milk to initiate and maintain her milk supply until she is with her baby again. Separation can happen for medical reasons, and while in Canada mothers usually have access to a lengthy maternity leave, increasingly mothers in other countries are required to return to work shortly after the birth of their babies in order to maintain their employment and earn an income. Regardless of the reasons for the separation of mom and baby, the intensity of expressing required to initiate and maintain a full milk supply is extreme, and it is often difficult to maintain. Information on how to pump can be hard to find and is not always accurate. Support from friends and family—and unfortunately sometimes even medical staff— can be lacking, making it all the more difficult to continue the efforts of pumping when away from your baby. Eventually, a mother's milk supply may decrease and the ability to breastfeed is compromised, or a baby may simply take so well to bottle-feeding that breastfeeding becomes a struggle and is no longer attempted.

Introduction of a Bottle

The introduction of a bottle is something that is rife with controversy. Some suggest there is no harm in it and others vehemently oppose the introduction of a bottle to a young baby arguing that artificial nipples, and the manner in which a baby sucks from a bottle, can interfere with a baby's ability to successfully nurse. This is not the place to pick sides or argue the case for or against, but it is certainly the place to discuss the introduction of bottles as a possible reason for breastfeeding failure.

There are many moms on both sides of the issue who can present their own opinions for or against bottle-feeding a breastfed baby. The key aspect here is to point out that for some mother-baby pairs, the introduction of a bottle, regardless of what is in the bottle, can be detrimental to the breastfeeding relationship. For some babies, a bottle may affect the way they suck. Some babies may become partial to the relative ease of flow from a bottle, particularly if they are having challenges breastfeeding effectively. For some mothers, bottles may be seen as an easier alternative during times of breastfeeding difficulty. In all cases, the introduction of a bottle can certainly interfere with the natural process of lactation and the ability of a baby to regulate a mother's supply as is done when a baby is allowed to feed on cue, or on demand. Many breastfed babies can successfully switch back and forth between bottle and breast, and many mothers have no choice but to bottle-feed their breastfed babies in order to facilitate their return to work, but although some moms and babies find success, others will find it leads to a negative outcome. Unfortunately, it's not always possible to predict which baby will have difficulties transitioning between the two.

Delivery Complications and Interventions

Birth is a natural process. As women, our bodies are amazing in their ability to nurture our babies within our wombs for nine months and then go through the birth process in order to continue nurturing our babes at our breast. Ina May Gaskin instructs women to "Remember this, for it is as true as true gets: Your body is not a lemon. You are not a machine. The Creator is not a careless mechanic. Human female bodies have the same potential to give birth well as aardvarks, lions, rhinoceri, elephants, moose, and water buffalo. Even if it has not been your habit throughout your life so far, I recommend that you learn to think positively about your body."[10] Our bodies are incredible in their power, strength, and nurturing abilities. However, the modern medical establishment's statistics on birth interventions and complications would not seem to support this idea. Close to one in four births in Canada are now c-sections and in the U.S. rates are over 31%.[11] Certainly this is not the type of birth experience we are intended to have.

Along with high c-section rates are extremely high rates of interventions which include: pitocin use, epidurals, fetal monitoring, forceps and vacuum extraction, episiotomies, separation of mom and baby following delivery, and various forms of pain management. All forms of interventions include some risk to the breastfeeding relationship. While most if not all effects can be overcome, it is not always easy to overcome them and without accurate information and strong support from professionals and friends and family, the challenges can sometimes prove too difficult to surmount.

Medical Reasons for Breastfeeding Failure

There are a number of medical conditions that can make breastfeeding more challenging. Often, expectant women who have these conditions are not told of the possibilities for complication of lactation, and they are left to attempt to sort out breastfeeding difficulties on their own, instead of having the opportunity to be proactive and take steps to limit the impact of these conditions. Conditions such as polycystic ovarian syndrome (PCOS), diabetes, and hypoplastic breasts (or insufficient glandular tissue) can impact milk supply making it more challenging to fully breastfeed. Even cigarette smoking and certain post-delivery complications have potential impacts on breastfeeding.

When women are not made aware of the possible effects caused by these conditions, they are again left to wade through the resulting challenges on their own, often feeling as though they have failed and have somehow been the cause of the breastfeeding difficulties. But in reality it is the three overriding elements first mentioned—lack of knowledge, lack of support, pressures from society—which are affecting women's ability to breastfeed. Even when breastfeeding is challenged by a medical condition, mothers can often find their own measure of success if lactation is planned and considered ahead of time.

We've now discussed how a lack of knowledge can affect breastfeeding, now let's consider how a lack of support can lead to negative consequences.

Lack of Support

Support—whether it be informational or emotional support—is essential for a new mother. Support comes from many different sources including support from medical professionals, friends, family, and society. In my personal experience, on the medical front, my family doctor informed me after my son had been home for only a couple of days that it was okay to "just feed formula". He had two children: one breastfed and one formula-fed, and there was, according to him, no difference between them. Another doctor, this time a paediatrician, couldn't get past the fact that I was, at that point in time, bottle-feeding my son but feeding expressed breast milk. He asked no fewer than four times if I was bottle-feeding or breastfeeding. Each time I explained I was bottle-feeding expressed breast milk. He would then ask the same question as though my answer just didn't make sense. It was this doctor who, after explaining to him that my son was screaming and thrashing after almost every feed and projectile vomiting several times a day, told me there was nothing to worry about and to call him if things got worse. I left not knowing how much worse things could get and wondering if

I wasn't getting support from my doctors, who *would* give me the support I so desperately needed?

Through a paediatric walk-in clinic (no, I never gave up looking for help) I was finally able to locate a doctor who took pity on me and suggested I try an over-the-counter antacid medication for my son. Within twenty-four hours I had a completely different baby. By this time though, my son was five months old and we were both well established in the routine of pumping and bottle-feeding. Had I received better information and better support would things have turned out differently? I can't say for sure, but I do know my level of stress and the feelings of failure I carried with me during that time would have been reduced. At least I was blessed to have the support of my family during this challenging time, but not every new mother can say this.

Influence of Family and Friends

One area that may be overlooked when trying to come to terms with breastfeeding difficulties and failure is the impact family and friends can have on the breastfeeding relationship between a mother and her new baby. Fathers, in fact, are extremely influential in ensuring a mother and her baby are successful in their nursing relationship.[12] Being surrounded by people who understand the value of your efforts is critical; you need people who will be cheerleaders and coaches, firm with you when you need them to be and caring and compassionate when you're having a hard time seeing your way through. Being surrounded by people who don't believe in the value of breastfeeding, who don't understand why it is so important to you, and who don't understand how a single bottle of formula or the early introduction of a pacifier might interfere with your efforts, can create an enormous barrier to achieving your goals. We all want to please those around us, and often when we are struggling it is easier to give in to the influence of friends and family members.

This isn't to say that friends and families don't want the best for us or our babies; they of course usually do, but with the constant misinformation directed at mothers, most people in our society have been socialised to believe that formula is the standard way to feed a baby—"I was formula-fed and there's nothing wrong with me!" During the height of difficulties or post-partum blues is not the time to try to stand your ground or educate those around you. Preparing your support group ahead of time, and educating those in your life about the importance of breastfeeding to you and your baby (and even on a larger scale the importance of breastfeeding to them and society at large) can help you avoid the negative results that can come about when friends and family are not supportive of your breastfeeding efforts. More about developing your support system will be discussed in an upcoming chapter.

The one thing I am thankful for is a supportive family. For the most part, everyone was very encouraging. My parents kindly offered to pay for the rental of the breast pump from the hospital, and no one within my family or group of friends ever suggested I switch to formula. They tolerated my need for a structured pumping schedule and never questioned why I was so determined to keep trying. My husband did have a few moments in which he questioned my insistence, but I think this came from a sense of powerlessness. He couldn't make it better for me. He couldn't do anything to make the stress or pain go away. He had no control and yet he, as most men would, felt the need to make the situation better for his wife. It was most definitely a trying time, but I realize that many new mothers are faced with much worse.

At Your Most Vulnerable

One of my biggest frustrations with regards to articles on breastfeeding is the fact that many discuss, at least to some extent, the negatives. They usually start out with how difficult and challenging it can be, followed by how painful it is, and then for good measure often throw in some aspect of it being a burden and time constraining. It's no wonder women who are expecting a child will say, "I'm going to *try* to breastfeed and see how it goes." Can there be hope for something that is presented in such a dismal light?

Granted, these challenges can arise (and given the fact you're reading this book, you've likely experienced some of them yourself), but they should not be the norm. Yet new mothers are set up to fail by being fed fear and negative emotions prior to the experience. If we fear something, we go into the experience already having a physical reaction to it. We might be tense or have a boost of adrenaline in our system. We expect the worst and often find our worst fears come true: a case of self-fulfilling prophecy.

Breastfeeding is no different. Breastfeeding your first baby is an experience no one can really prepare you for, and yet what you read about it prepares you for an experience that surely must be difficult and likely painful and most definitely time-consuming. We may be surrounded by other women who have had less than wonderful breastfeeding experiences and their emotions are often transferred to us. My mother kept telling me how painful it was when her baby started biting—that's when she weaned! Women like to do the same thing when it comes to childbirth; we hear the horror stories and rarely the wonderful experiences.

While this might not be a common reason given for breast-feeding difficulties, I think it is a valid one, and it is likely more common than we realize. Hidden behind pain, fatigue, low milk supply, and early supplementation may very well be fear and other negative emotions: fear of the unknown, fear of mother-hood, fear of being totally responsible for a precious little life, fear of not doing *it* well. It's not the fault of new mothers, and it perhaps isn't something that can be easily controlled, but it is there.

Pressures from Society

Fear may be stoked by family and friends, but it may also be a result of the broader experiences we have in our society. Society's impact on our lives as new mothers is ever-present and its impact on me as a new mother, a new mother struggling with breastfeeding, was immense. Formula companies sent lovely packages with full-sized samples of their products and significant discount coupons. A walk through any local store reminded me that there was another option to breastfeeding: one as easy as picking up a can of formula off the shelf and walking to the cashier—oh, and don't forget the $10.00 off coupon. Bottles and gadgets lined up on the store shelves promised a solution to the problems I was trying hard to overcome. Pregnancy and parenting magazines dropped tantalizing marketing campaigns into my mailbox, again assuring me that the path I was trying so hard to follow was not the only way. While these magazines often included articles on how to breastfeed, the advertising from formula companies contained within their pages reduced the benefit those articles provided. Indeed all the mothers in the advertising looked well-rested, free of stress, and able to care for their perfect babies. What was I doing continuing to struggle to breastfeed?

Sometimes family members do not support the breastfeeding efforts of a new mother. The old argument of "I wasn't breastfed and I turned out okay" gets thrown around and is sometimes used to convince a new mother that she should wean and switch to formula. Maybe this comes from the human need to believe we are doing what is best for our children, but I think the influence of society is at play not only in our own lives but in the lives of those around us: our mothers and aunts and grandmothers whose society encouraged them to embrace advancement and science and bottle-feed baby formula.

Women my mother's age were told to put their faith in science and formula companies, told that indeed science had surpassed nature and was capable of producing a product to feed our infants that was just as good as, if not better than, mother's milk. But how could this claim be believed? In hindsight, it would seem that science and medicine do not always know what is best. My husband's grandmother was told in the 1950s to start smoking cigarettes in order to calm her nerves. Her doctor told her it would be *good* for her. Thankfully, our understanding of breastfeeding—and smoking—is much better today and breastfeeding is returning to its appropriate place, but it is easy to understand the need some women might feel to justify the decision they made years ago, especially in the face of the new research available. Recognizing where your family and friends are coming from and understanding the experiences that they bring with them, will help you to make wise choices when it comes to the support you receive from the people around you and from society in general. Unfortunately, family, friends, and society aren't always supportive and this can have a great impact on your efforts to work through breastfeeding difficulties and come out successfully on the other side.

In the end, I wasn't successful breastfeeding my first baby. I ended up exclusively pumping breast milk for my son for a year. True, he received my milk, but still at the time I felt that I had failed. Crazy when you consider how much I did in order for my son to have breast milk for his first year. Did I fail? No way! But this realization has come only with the passing of years. Don't let years pass before you come to this realization for yourself.

∾∾∾

The Comfort of Numbers

Often you will hear a new mother say of bottle-feeding: "I like the fact that I know how much my baby is eating." And indeed it is true. When using a bottle to feed a baby, whether it be formula or breast milk in the bottle, you have the peace of mind of knowing your baby is getting a certain amount of food. In fact, this is often one of the positives formula companies offer when comparing the benefits of breastfeeding and formula feeding. However, this reliance on numbers—the comfort one feels knowing how much a baby is eating and the comfort a woman can feel knowing just how much milk she is producing—can also serve to make it more difficult to transition to exclusive breastfeeding.

When my son was born nine weeks premature, he began a five-week stay in the neonatal intensive care unit (NICU) and his hospital stay was centred around numbers—numbers dealing with, of course, his weight, but particularly numbers dealing with his feeding. The very first things we were usually told on our daily visits to the NICU were how much milk our son was now receiving through his nasogastric tube (NG tube) and how much weight he had gained. His feeding schedule was also always reported to us as a sign that he was getting stronger and able to eat more at longer intervals: q2 and then q3 and then home!

When I started attempting to breastfeed, numbers were never far from me. After only a couple of attempts, the nurse had me start pre and post weights to quantify just how much my son was taking at the breast and determine how much more he needed through his NG tube. For the two weeks prior to his release, I stayed at the hospital with my son and focused on establishing a successful breastfeeding relationship. *Prior* to every feed I would weigh him and record the numbers. *After* every feed I would weigh him and record the numbers. Throughout this time I was *also* religiously recording the volume of each pumping session to determine just how my milk supply was doing. I was keeping records as a means to prove to myself, and to others, that things were going as they should be, or that things were not working out as well as hoped. I became a slave to these records.

Mothers of full-term babies are not immune to this numbers game. So many mothers are urged to supplement with a bottle soon after the birth of their baby. The suggestion is usually presented as a baby's need for food since a mother's milk may not yet have come in. When the normal breastfeeding pattern of a newborn is to nurse frequently but for short periods of time, it is easy to be lead to believe that you do not have the milk necessary to satisfy your baby. And when you see your baby take a couple ounces by bottle and can quantify your baby's intake and know that you are providing food, it is easy to become misguided and start to question your ability to provide sufficient breast milk for your baby. However, your baby, in its instinctual wisdom, knows best, and, indeed, this frequent nursing is the best thing to establish a strong supply of breast milk.

Of course supplementation with formula means that a baby is not stimulating the breast as frequently, a mother is not removing as much milk as possible, and a mother's milk supply may very well start to diminish. This can lead to an unhappy baby who is not being satisfied at the breast since milk production has declined. A baby may start to balk at the breast, refuse the breast, fuss at the breast, fall asleep at the breast, and any other number of reactions. Of course a mother, wanting only to see her new baby satisfied, turns to the bottle feeling relieved knowing her baby is eating sufficient amounts.

Supplementation soon after birth is, of course, not the only reason a baby may be bottle-fed. Difficulties establishing breastfeeding can also force a mother to use a bottle to supplement breastfeeding attempts. In this situation as well, there is comfort knowing that even though you continue to work at establishing a successful breastfeeding relationship, you are able to ensure your baby is eating well. And indeed sometimes the reduced stress involved with bottle-feeding (as opposed to the screaming and thrashing and kicking and crying—of both mother and baby—that can come with difficulties breastfeeding) can make the bottle a refuge and a comfortable shelter from the stress and anxiety surrounding the attempts to nourish your baby at the breast.

The problem with the numbers that naturally come with bottle-feeding and expressing breast milk is that they become a comfort and a means of control. When breastfeeding, you have no numbers other than the frequency and length of time your baby is feeding. You have no idea how much your baby is receiving. Your only indication is the assurance that your baby is growing and gaining weight. But when bottle-feeding and expressing milk, you have the ability to monitor your baby's intake and your output. You can see your milk in front of you, lined up in the fridge or packed into the freezer. It is tangible. To switch from pumping your breast milk and feeding it with a bottle to exclusively breastfeeding requires a large leap of faith and a belief that your baby knows how to regulate your supply and will nurse efficiently at the breast, and a belief that your body will continue to produce milk. This leap of faith is a major obstacle that prevents many mothers from transitioning their babies to exclusive breastfeeding after they have been exclusively pumping or using formula supplementation in addition to nursing.

Now there are of course situations in which a baby just does not get the hang of breastfeeding or isn't physically capable of breastfeeding, but there are also many situations in which a baby will latch but perhaps does not nurse consistently every time. In these situations, there is often an opportunity to place your trust in your baby and roll the dice, so to speak. And it *is* a roll of the dice in some respects. To switch to exclusive breastfeeding means that you will no longer be pumping, and pumping has likely been the one thing over which you have had some degree of control. To switch to exclusive breastfeeding means that you will not be scheduling when your baby feeds or when you empty your breasts, but you will instead need to allow your baby to nurse on request. To switch to exclusive breastfeeding means that you will not have the comfort of your daily record of pumping volumes or your baby's daily intake; you will need to believe that things are as they need to be. And even if you do manage to put your faith in your baby's ability, there is no guarantee things will work out. Your baby might just not be able to transfer enough milk; he might continue to be fussy at the breast even when allowed to nurse as often as desired; you might feel as though your supply is starting to diminish if your baby is not nursing well; and you might find that the stress of trying to transition over to exclusive breastfeeding is just too much to bear and that you would rather have your baby content and the stress of breastfeeding removed from your life.

But you may just find that your baby does know what he is doing and that you do establish a successful breastfeeding relationship. And in the opinion of many, this would be a wonderful thing. It is a risk in some ways and frightening in some ways, and, in the end, the decision to take the plunge and attempt to transition to exclusive breastfeeding is in your hands.

When I was in the early months of exclusively pumping, I had to struggle with many of these issues. Once my son was home from the hospital, I became obsessed with the numbers. I had built such a reliance in the hospital on the pre and post weights to determine how my son was feeding, I had no knowledge of how to tell if he was breastfeeding well or not. I did, however, know how much milk he took from his bottle. I always knew exactly how much I was pumping. I had a written record to prove my success.

There was a brief window of time, when I look back, during which I may have been able to transition to breastfeeding exclusively. But the fear of the unknown and the loss of control I felt at not having those daily numbers in front of me held me back. I worried that I would lose my supply if I stopped pumping for a few days and relied only on my son to maintain my supply (naïve perhaps, but the fear was very real for me at that point). I worried that if breastfeeding didn't work out, I would not go back to pumping and my son would instead have to be fed formula. I felt it better that he received breast milk, regardless of how it was delivered, than receive formula. This, of course, is not the only reason I continued to exclusively pump, but it certainly did factor into my decision not to jump in with both feet—if only for a day or two—and see if my son could exclusively breastfeed.

When I weaned, I gathered the notebooks in which I had recorded all my pumping sessions (yes, I had more than one notebook), and I started to calculate the quantity of breast milk I had expressed and the amount of time I spent expressing breast milk over that year. In total, I had pumped approximately 389 litres of milk and spent approximately one entire month expressing that milk. Those numbers were, and still are, staggering to me. Those numbers, in many ways, encapsulate the year I exclusively pumped. And yet, they were a burden to me. They were a reminder of my inability to breastfeed and a symbol of my obsession to provide breast milk for my son. I am immensely proud of myself for pumping when breastfeeding did not turn out as expected, and I feel even more strongly now that breast milk is the absolute best way to nourish an infant and that exclusively pumping should be presented to all mothers who are unable to breastfeed as a viable alternative to formula. But I also recognize how my actions were driven by a need within me to "do this right", and in some way, make up for the loss of a breastfeeding relationship with my son. The numbers in my notebooks were a means of controlling my experience and a way to cope with the loss of what I had expected to experience.

Six months after I weaned, I threw those notebooks away. In some ways, I wish I hadn't even kept them at all. But when I did throw them away, I also threw away all the grief and guilt and sadness I felt over not being able to breastfeed my son — although I still hang on to a little bit of regret. The numbers in those notebooks meant nothing. What was meaningful was the love and dedication that allowed me to fill those notebooks. It didn't matter that breastfeeding had not worked out as expected but that I did what I needed to do for my son given the situation that was handed to us.

Breastfeeding, Take Two

Do You Think I'm Guilty?

"I was angry and defensive and was ashamed to be seen giving
him a bottle."

Laura, mother of two

Mommy guilt. It's unavoidable. Every new mother feels it. It creeps in uninvited sometime during the first few weeks of your baby's life. It is ever-present, and in many ways, it is a sign that you are a good mother. Guilt is a signal that you love your child; you want to do everything you possibly can for your child. You want to give them the best. Who can fault you for that? But when the feeling of guilt and worry—the belief that you are somehow harming your child— begins to overwhelm you or becomes all consuming or ever-present, mommy guilt has reached a whole new level.

A mother who experiences difficulties with breastfeeding often becomes consumed with this sense of guilt: a belief that she has let her baby down, that she has not given everything she could to her baby. Guilt is the name women will commonly give to the emotion they are feeling. Diane Wiessinger, in her essay "The Language of Breastfeeding", points the finger directly at a system that isn't doing what it needs to do saying, "'We don't want to make bottle-feeding mothers feel angry. We don't want to make them feel betrayed. We don't want to make them feel cheated.' Peel back the layered implications of 'we don't want to make them feel guilty,' and you will find a system trying to cover its own tracks. It is not trying to protect her. It is trying to protect itself. Let's level with mothers, support them when breastfeeding doesn't work, and help them move beyond this inaccurate and ineffective word."[1] But is it really guilt? Do we really feel guilty when we fail at breastfeeding?

In most cases, what women are feeling is more accurately described as grief rather than guilt. Guilt is something we feel when we know we could have done more, but didn't. When we went against our better judgement and made a choice we knew wasn't the best for those involved. Or when we blatantly make a decision that we know is only in our own best interest and not in the best interest of those who we are to care for and love. Do some women feel guilty when they do not breastfeed? Most definitely yes. But this is based on making a decision that they know is not right for their baby and yet moving forward with it. This guilt certainly can be overwhelming and impact a woman's decision to breastfeed another child, but more central to our discussion here is the experience of women who desperately wanted to breastfeed, did everything they could to make it work, and are not able to find success. For these women, while guilt may often be the word used to describe their feelings, grief is perhaps a more accurate one.

The distinction between guilt and grief is not based on the amount of effort you put into breastfeeding or the length of time you persevered. It really has more to do with the information you had at the time, your efforts to access information and support, and your dedication to do everything you could do *at the time*. Once you have exhausted your resources—and for some, those resources are going to be very thin—you have a decision to make. If you are faced with a baby who is hungry, who is not gaining weight, or who is crying incessantly, you need to feed your baby. Without the resources and support to help you breastfeed successfully, what else are you going to choose? You choose to bottle-feed. For some women this means expressing milk and feeding milk in a bottle (exclusively pumping), and for other women this means switching their baby to artificial baby milk, or formula. When you have exhausted your resources, and done all you can do, there is no reason to feel guilty. As new mothers, we do what we believe is right at the time. There is no guilt in that.

On a very personal level, I understand this sense of guilt all too well. When my son was born so early and so tiny, the guilt set in. My body had failed him. I had developed preeclampsia at thirty weeks and he was showing signs of intrauterine growth restriction. The day before I was induced, doctors tested the umbilical blood flow and determined that it was in the ninety-seventh percentile. This high percentile was not a good thing and meant the blood flow in the cord was compromised. My son was doing okay, but my body was quickly shutting down and the doctors said that he had to be delivered right away. My determination was then to ensure I could breastfeed. I remember asking several times during a quick tour of the NICU what the likelihood of breastfeeding was going to be. Would I be able to breastfeed my son? All indications were positive and so I clung to that hope. My body wouldn't fail my son again.

But five weeks later, even though my son was doing very well with expressed milk and I was determined to make breastfeeding work, it was not working. Feelings of failure were strong; I figured I just didn't know what I was doing. The lactation consultants in the hospital seemed frustrated that my son was not breastfeeding better than he was, and I internalized this frustration thinking I was the cause. As I left the hospital for the first time with my son, I remember feeling emotionally numb. I was operating largely on auto-pilot and still clinging to the belief—the hope—that breastfeeding was going to work out.

Of course, life never goes as planned and things got progressively worse at home. Eventually, it got to the point where he was projectile vomiting several times a day, screaming after most feedings, and thrashing and wailing if I attempted to latch him. It became very personal. Was my son rejecting me? I sought out assistance from lactation consultants and breastfeeding experts. The advice ranged from "It's okay to switch to formula if that is what you want" to "You've got to get that baby to the breast" but with no offer of help or useful suggestions. Of course as mentioned previously in the book, after finally resigning myself to exclusively pumping, partly to preserve at least a small amount of my sanity and partly as a retreat from defeat, I found one doctor who offered the suggestion of using a readily available, over-the-counter medicine to see if perhaps it might help my son. In less than twenty-four hours it was as though a new baby had moved into the house.

Guilt? You bet! But I quickly realized that I had done everything I could do with what I was given. I had lactation support in the hospital. I sought out lactation support when my son was released from the hospital. I talked to my doctor. I demanded a referral to a paediatrician. I read the books. I searched online. I was screaming for help; and yet the system failed me. What more could I have done? Could I have continued trying to breastfeed exclusively? Possibly. But anyone who has every gone through the cycle of breastfeeding, pumping, and bottle-feeding understands what an incredible toll that takes on you. It is not a long-term solution. Could I have stopped pumping and just breastfed to see just how well my son would have done if he was forced to breastfeed with no bottle in sight? I could have, but I felt at the time that all I had going for me was a strong milk supply and feared that I might risk it all if I stopped pumping. I felt alone and lonely in the experience. And in hindsight, I know that I did all I could do, physically and emotionally, to make it work. But still it didn't.

And so we're left with guilt and grief. Once you work through the feelings of guilt, and recognize that you have done all you could do given your knowledge, support, and physical and emotional limitations, you are left with the grief. Breastfeeding is a biologically expected activity. It is, for most women, a relationship that is deeply desired. To lose that relationship is to lose something very real, something that has value and purpose and meaning. Just as we mourn when we lose a person we love, we must also mourn the loss of the relationship we wished for.

Part of the challenge in understanding these feelings as grief, as opposed to guilt, is the way that breastfeeding is framed in our society. Many people surrounding you may have a "get over it" attitude. Many suggest to new moms who are having breast-feeding difficulties, "Just switch to formula." But these attitudes and well-intended suggestions serve only to make us feel that our emotions are wrong and that feeling sad over our loss is invalid—but they most definitely are not! Working through these emotions is critical, both to your well-being and your baby's well-being. Coming to terms with your shared, rocky start will help you grow and move forward.

Guilt, Grief, and Future Babies

Regardless of what we call it—guilt, grief, or regret—the experience of losing the breastfeeding relationship you had hoped for and expected can, and most likely will, affect you in the future. It may hide in a corner or be an obvious stumbling block in your decision to have other children. It may appear to have been tamed and controlled, only to unleash itself when you get that positive sign on the pregnancy test. The impact of breastfeeding failure can be varied, but for most women who experienced difficulties breastfeeding a first baby, the impact is very real.

Speaking about this feeling of failure, Laura states, "I was devastated and felt, very starkly, that I had failed my son. I was angry and defensive and was ashamed to be seen giving him a bottle. I was furious, too, that I couldn't pump enough milk to nourish him exclusively on breast milk. I avoided conversations about nursing at all costs." The progression of sadness and grief to anger is normal, and it is this progression of emotions and states of mind that can be used to help move you past the tragedy of the experience and towards a better outcome the next time around.

During the three years between having my son and staring at the positive pregnancy test announcing the impending arrival of my daughter, I thought I had sufficiently dealt with the impact of a failed breastfeeding attempt. The loss of expectations was what hit me the most: the expected normal labour, the expected easy breastfeeding, the expected closeness breastfeeding would bring with my son. Expectations are dangerous things, especially when it comes to things over which we have little control! I exclusively pumped for a year, so my son still had most of the benefits of breastfeeding. I wrote a book about exclusively pumping and worked through many of the lingering emotions I had about my experience during the writing process. My husband and I had weighed the considerable risks of another pregnancy and the risk of preeclampsia occurring a second time. I thought I was pre-pared—until the reality of a new pregnancy hit me.

I would have expected to be worried about developing pre-eclampsia again. Having a baby at thirty-one weeks gestation with the stress and worries that go along with that is not some-thing anyone would wish to experience again. Yet when faced with the prospect of another baby, preeclampsia was the furthest thing from my mind. Instead, the first thought after the initial, *oh my*, was, *am I going to be able to breastfeed this baby*? What for most expectant mothers is at best an afterthought—or a few-months-afterthought—was the first thought on my mind. It began to consume me. The thought of not being able to breastfeed my second child was not something I even wanted to consider, and yet, I knew the reality was that it was something I had to consider. Why was it so paralysing? And why do many second-time moms feel the same way if they have been unable to breastfeed their first child? There are a few possible reasons.

Fear is a big one. Fear can be absolutely immobilising. Fearing failure can cause us simply not to make the attempt. Somewhere in our heads we know that not to try simply because we are afraid of failing is no excuse. We would certainly tell our children that you must try even if you do end up failing. It's better to try and fail, than to never try at all. Failure teaches us; it helps us learn and grow. As Samuel Beckett urged: "Try again. Fail again. Fail better." This is all well and good, but when faced with the fear, and the knowledge of what failure brings with it, choosing simply not to make the attempt might seem like a better option. And for some, it may be. But trying again can also be very healing and liberating.

The second time around you have much more experience and information. If you have considered your first breastfeeding attempt, you will hopefully have a good understanding of what failed you: lack of information, lack of support, societal pressures. You will hopefully have worked through the grief of your lost breastfeeding relationship with your first child and understand the myriad of ways you were able to develop the strong relationship with that child you undoubtedly have today. You will have an understanding that it is not all or nothing. Success can be determined by you alone and not others. You can set your goals and work towards reaching them. But all this can only happen if you move past the fear and take the step forward to trying it again.

What can be harder to move past is the learned belief that you are incapable of breastfeeding, that your body is flawed, or that you simply can't do it. This lie is being told to us over and over again through advertising, by our medical professionals, and is even being perpetuated by other women. But the fact of the matter is that our bodies do work—*your* body does work—we need to believe in it and trust it to do what it is meant to do and learn to ignore the onslaught of false information, and lack of information about breastfeeding, that is found in our society. We, as women, need to recognize the difference between normal newborn behaviour and normal *formula-fed* newborn behaviour and realize that those are two very different things. The information being presented about breastfeeding by family, friends, media, and sometimes even medical professionals, is too often accurate only for babies being fed artificial baby milk, and when we try to impose those schedules, expectations, and timelines on our breastfed babies, it's no wonder we face challenges, difficulties, and yes, even failure.

Gina from *The Feminist Breeder Blog* discusses this lie as it is being told. Referring to statistics from the Centers for Disease Control (CDC) in the United States that show three-quarters of women in the United States initiate breastfeeding in the hospital but only 13.6% are breastfeeding at six months post-partum, Gina declares, "Here is the cold hard truth, ladies: You have been lied to." Gina goes on to say

> If only 13.6% of us could make enough milk, the human race would never have survived. And it's not your fault. It's the fault of this system that completely fails mothers and babies, and sabotages a mother's good intentions. Somewhere along the line, someone told you that you couldn't make milk, and you believed them because we've all grown up in a culture that tells women their bodies aren't good enough for much of anything except

being toys for men. Is it easy to make this milk? No, not always—but neither was bringing that baby into the world and your body did a fine job of that. Think about that. Think hard. Your body created an entire human being inside from nothing more than the joining of two single cells. Your body is a miracle worker. So what leads you to believe that, after creating a whole person with organs and tissue and a beating heart, that your body would call it quits when it came time to feeding this thing?[2]

This lack of faith in our own bodies when it comes to breastfeeding is a continuation of the lies we are told during pregnancy and childbirth. With c-section rates in the United States reaching 32%[3] and most other countries following closely behind, women are increasingly led to believe that it is the medical establishment that delivers babies, not ourselves or our bodies. When I talk to friends and acquaintances, it is rare to hear a birth story that does not include some type of intervention: inductions, pitocin, pain control, monitoring, vacuum or forceps, episiotomies, c-sections. Is it any wonder after going through such an experience as this to birth our children that we would so easily accept that our bodies are also flawed when it comes to nourishing our children?

This obstacle can be more of a challenge to move past. Since this lack of faith in our bodies has taken time to develop, it can also take time to overcome. Education and connections with a support system are important tools in reacquiring—or perhaps acquiring for the first time — that faith we need to have in our bodies. Seek out positive birth stories and breastfeeding stories. Read books that strengthen your trust in yourself. Talk to friends about the myths and lies that we are told and try to establish new beliefs. Locate groups in your community that encourage and support a more normal view of pregnancy, childbirth, and breastfeeding. This doesn't mean you need to become an "earth mother" or a vegetarian or that you must use cloth diapers instead of disposable; what it means is that you are considering the narratives being told to us in our society, seeking out the truth, and debunking the myths. You can stop feeling guilty for not being able to breastfeed and instead recognize it for what it was, and move forward into your new pregnancy armed with knowledge and power, knowing that if for some reason things still don't go the way you hope the second time around, you have done everything you can to make it happen. And you can be sure that, with increased knowledge, your chances of success are also greatly increased.

But what if you are determined *not* to try again? What if you can work past the fear, recognise your body's inherent strengths, and yet still you do not want to try, feeling it would be better to skip the entire stage and move right to bottle-feeding? Are you perhaps feeling that since your first child wasn't breastfed, or breastfed as long as you planned, and they turned out fine, that there is no reason to put yourself through the possible stress, pain, and frustration a second time? Are you worried about giving something to one child that the other didn't get? This sense of robbing your child of something when you are not able to breastfeed is very common. In *Unbuttoned*, Jessica Restaino explains her sense of guilt and fear of taking something from her child saying, "Inside I felt only the heat of a guilty secret, a knowing sense that somehow I had cheated my baby. My mind swirled with blame: I had taken the easy way out."[4] While a sense of guilt over robbing your child of something may be common, you cannot let it affect your decisions with your next baby.

It's natural to want to give to your children equally, but is it fair? Look deep inside yourself and question the value you place on breastfeeding. Is it something worth doing? Is it the right thing, the normal thing, for a baby? If yes, then it is the right thing for *your* baby, regardless of whether your other child has been breastfed or not. It can be difficult knowing that one of our children has missed out on something. That one has been given benefits over the other. But it's also important to remember that we do our best for each of our children at the time. Breastfeeding aside, you are likely going to have many situations in which you handle things differently from one child to another child. With the first, you might give him or her more time, read more stories, ensure he or she eats a better diet. When the second child comes along, time fills up, and the second child might not get the same one-on-one time with you or may not enjoy new clothes as often as the first. Many things in life don't work out equally, but what is important is giving each child what they need when you are able to provide it. Your first child will recognize your love and dedication to them and will benefit from witnessing the breast-feeding relationship between you and your other child. While they might not have experienced it first-hand, they will witness it every day and understand the love you have for your children through your actions and nurturing ways. This is true whether you are breastfeeding or not.

Moving On

Moving forward and creating a new, different breastfeeding experience with a new baby requires a few things be done. First, it is important to take some time to reflect on what was expected the first time around. What expectations did you have for the process of breastfeeding? How were those expectations met or not met? It's natural to have expectations about things, but having expectations without flexibility can lead to an increased sense of loss. When you only picture one possible outcome, there is nothing but disappointment and loss from any other outcome. And so take the opportunity to consider what you expect, how you will react if those expectations are not met, and how alterations to those expectations will affect your breastfeeding journey. Once you have done this, spend some time considering what was lost when those original expectations were not met.

When breastfeeding doesn't go as expected, there is a true loss for both mother and baby. As mothers, we lose out on what we planned for and hoped for, and both we and our babies lose the natural process and bonding relationship fostered by breastfeeding. It is so important to recognize it as a loss and allow yourself to grieve the loss. It's okay, normal even, to be sad. Often those around us don't recognize the loss or understand why we feel so sad. If you're feeling overwhelmed and have no one to talk to, consider finding a doctor or therapist to whom you can voice your emotions. Do not bottle up your feelings, or push them away thinking that you're overreacting. It is sad when a mother and baby lose the opportunity for a nursing relationship, and working through your emotions will help you put your experience in perspective and shore up your strength to try again.

The next important step is to recognize the experience for what it was. Everything we do is a learning experience. We don't always have all the answers; no one expects us to. But we do have the opportunity to learn from our experience and move forward with intention. Once you're feeling capable of honestly looking at the reasons breastfeeding didn't work out, try to pinpoint what it was that went wrong. Consider the three big elements discussed earlier in the book: lack of information, lack of support, and societal pressures and influence. Where did it go wrong in your case? Be clear here. This is not intended to be a blame game. The idea isn't to find blame in what you did or didn't do. We all do the best we can, with the information we have, at a given time. But to move forward, we need to be able to look critically at our experiences and actions and understand what happened.

The grief you feel is deeply personal and is something that you alone need to work through. Jessica Restaino considers this personal aspect of grief and breastfeeding explaining, "In many ways that's what getting better was like. It was a breaking away from something deeply personal, deeply mine."[5] This "deeply personal" aspect of breastfeeding is felt by almost every mother. It's our biology that creates it and yet it's our culture that defines it. If our society tells women that they are being ridiculous for being so emotional over not breastfeeding, then mothers are left feeling badly about the sadness and grief. Restaino states that her "sadness became a source of guilt."[6] It is so important to recognize your emotions for what they are: sadness, grief, anger, guilt...whatever it may be. Accept it as your own, work through it, and then, most importantly, figure out a way to move past it.

Once you've grieved the loss and examined your experience and hopefully better understand what happened, the last steps are to reframe your experience in a positive way and then move forward with intention. While you may never look back on your breastfeeding difficulties with fondness, they are part of your story, your experience. They have added to the person you are today. Perhaps your experience has given you greater empathy, encouraged you to search out new ways to bond with your baby, or brought you new friends you may not otherwise have met. Your difficulties have certainly helped you understand the level of your own persistence and drive, as well as your own limitations. Considering what you have gained, and not just what was lost, can help you move forward with purpose and renewed commitment.

Then, with a positive focus, you can set your intentions for your breastfeeding relationship with your new baby. Intentions are powerful things. Miriam-Webster online dictionary defines "intentions" as: "a determination to act in a certain way," and "what one intends to do or bring about."[7] I think the first definition is most interesting in this discussion. It's impossible to control what happens to us in life. Sometimes, things just happen. We don't expect them or plan for them, but we can control our reaction to them. Moving forward from your first breastfeeding experience, you may not be able to control your birth experience, or whether your new baby is eager to latch, but you can set your intentions for how you act in a given situation.

Moving forward with intention includes preparing and planning so you will have the resources and support you need if your experience throws you a curveball. If your baby doesn't latch right away, do you have the phone number of a competent, certified lactation consultant and the knowledge of when you need to start expressing your milk? If your baby wants to nurse seemingly all the time, do you have a support system in place to help you cope with these demands, encourage you to persevere, as well as knowledgeable people around you to help you know when there may be a problem? And if you are unsure what a normal nursing pattern is for a five-day-old baby, will you have the resources to determine the answer instead of caving in to the pressures of family telling you to use formula to "top up" the baby? Considering these kinds of questions before you have another baby will ensure you have the skills, knowledge, and support in place to move forward with intention and fulfill those intentions.

It's easy to point out the ways we feel we have let our children down: things that we didn't do, should have done, or did but shouldn't have. Mommy guilt. This is always going to be part of motherhood. So you weren't able to breastfeed your first baby. That is a terrible loss, and one that you need to grieve and move forward from, but it's not the sum total of your value as a mother. Remember to keep it all in perspective. You love your baby. You do everything you can to give your child the best possible in every area. Sometimes as parents we don't do so great, and other times, we are awesome. This is life. Breastfeeding is just another aspect of mothering. It's worth fighting for, and is wonderful when it works out, but it does not define you as a mother, nor does it define your relationship with your child.

When working through your breastfeeding loss, and preparing to move forward into a breastfeeding relationship with a new baby, take some time to also remember all the things you did, and do, for your baby. The fact you attempted to breastfeed shows your care. Your determination and persistence to try and make it work shows your love. Your willingness to push through the pain and discomfort testifies to your dedication to your child. If you did all you could given your circumstances, then there is no room for guilt. Regret, yes. But not guilt. Grieve, move on, learn from your experience, and prepare for a new experience with intention.

Flora's Story

Before becoming pregnant, I always thought I would breastfeed for six months minimum. It never even entered my mind that breastfeeding might be something I wouldn't be able to do. I knew that breast milk gave babies the best start, and I wanted that bonding experience as well. During pregnancy I was told by my sister to start brushing my nipples with a soft, gentle brush of some sort to "toughen them up". I tried once and it felt uncomfortable, and I started to wonder if I would have problems if I didn't toughen them up. My first background worries started then. I did, however, expect breastfeeding to be a wonderful, natural, beautiful time with my child. Almost picture perfect.

When my daughter was born by unplanned c-section, I was very dozy from drugs and did not feel safe to even hold her, let alone be in charge of her. But my husband and I were wheeled to an initial room and left alone to care for my daughter. When she fussed, about an hour and a half after birth, I asked the nurse if I should try nursing. I felt totally out of my depth and unsure of what to do. The nurse confirmed I should try, and I did with some success. I was in hospital for three days, feeling totally overwhelmed and unprepared for my responsibilities. My daughter wouldn't sleep on her back and was even inconsistent with sleeping on her side. She did, however, snuggle right into daddy's chest and sleep peacefully.

I felt incompetent not being able to settle my child myself. Hormones were rampant! Over the three days in hospital my daughter would clamp her jaw down during nursing and cause considerable pain. I was told by one nurse that my positioning was fine, and that pain was normal. Another nurse told me I should have no pain and to alter my positioning. Nothing helped. I was discharged having given approval for the public health nurse to phone me.

The next day, after a sleepless night due to plenty of crying (by both babe and mom) and feeling very unsettled, the public health nurse phoned, and I practically begged her to come to my house. She came out and said that my daughter's weight was fine, to try manually expressing some milk, and to alter my positioning. She also offered me a breastfeeding buddy, which I declined at the time. She came several times that first week and then my file was to be closed as they are only to visit a few times. She was very understanding though, and did try to help. She recommended seeing a lactation consultant, which we did. The lactation consultant told us that my let-down was so strong that my daughter was getting too much milk too quickly and in effect, drowning in it. In order to control the flow, she was clamping down. I was told to manually express and try different positions, but no follow-up was suggested.

I went home and manually expressed my milk, which did not help. My nipples were bleeding from open areas at the base (I now have scars there). I was in so much pain that I had to hold my breath and usually scream to get my daughter on my breast. She was really fussy (small wonder when someone screams when you're trying to eat). This was all within the first two weeks home.

I felt like an utter failure. My sister and mother encouraged me to formula feed, saying that I had given it my best shot and not to beat myself up and to move on. The public health nurse tried one more thing, a nipple shield, for nursing while also pumping to ease the painful nipples. My daughter didn't take to the nipple shield well, and I was so deflated by this point I wanted to stop. I did pump for another two weeks and bottle-feed her expressed milk, and then I just moved to formula, with so much guilt. I felt I was letting my daughter down, and even my husband. I felt that I had failed miserably at the two things that only I was supposed to be able to do for my baby—give birth and breastfeed.

The entire breastfeeding experience left me feeling like a failure. I became depressed. My husband wanted to have more children fairly quickly (two years apart), but I didn't feel I could do that. I didn't think I would be able to handle it.

Should I be blessed with another child, I would want to try breastfeeding again. I would definitely enlist some support around me. I didn't have good support the first time. I did in the end ask for the breastfeeding buddy to call, and I felt that she was not very open or understanding, just hostile and judgmental about my troubles. I never contacted her again.

Breastfeeding, Take Two

The Best-Laid Plans

"I was slapped in the face by reality—this was not part of my birth plan and things were not going the way I had envisioned them."

Heather, mom of two

T hink back to your first pregnancy. What did you do to prepare for the arrival of your first child? What did you read, watch, and buy? What were your expectations and plans? Did you have a birth plan? Did you have expectations for how things would be? If you are like most expectant new mothers you read books such as *What to Expect When You're Expecting*, watched television shows such as *A Baby Story*, and read some of the many magazines aimed at expectant mothers.

Pregnancy is a time of expectation and excitement. That is after all why it is referred to as "expecting." We are expecting an enjoyable pregnancy, a healthy baby, a good birth experience, and a close breastfeeding relationship. But reality does not always meet our expectations, and when this happens it can be difficult and sometimes devastating to acknowledge the reality of the situation and accept what is, instead of what was hoped for.

Dangerous Expectations

There is a myriad of stories told to us as pregnant women. Some of these stories suggest pregnancy and childbirth are lovely, wonderful, joyous, memorable experiences. Some of these stories suggest pregnancy and childbirth are experiences of pain, medicalization, and intervention; a healthy baby is all that matters; and breastfeeding is a difficult proposition, often painful, and that not all women can breastfeed. The odd thing about life is that we tend to get what we expect.

This truth has been popularized in recent years with the publication of *The Secret* and discussions about the power of positive thinking, but it really isn't new or surprising. This reality became apparent to me as a child when I was learning to ride a horse and was told to look where I wanted to go. If you look elsewhere, the horse will go elsewhere. Should we be surprised that we tend to get what we expect or achieve what we set our sights on in life? "Keep your eyes on the prize" is another popular expression which suggests the same idea.

During pregnancy, we also make plans and create expectations; we focus our attention on the events to come and consider how we would like them to unfold. However, the messages we receive from our culture, our society, our friends and family, popular media, and a range of other sources, affect how we develop our vision and expectations. There is also a dissonance between what we may include in a birth plan; the reality of what is possible given the practices, protocols, and realities of a hospital birth; and the messages we are receiving about childbirth and breastfeeding. You may verbalize your intentions to breastfeed, but the messages from society and friends about the pain and difficulty of breastfeeding may in fact over-ride all your positive intentions. This gulf between what we intend to do and what we are told creates a division within us that makes the realization of our intentions much more challenging. This affects not only our desires to breastfeed but also affects us much earlier in our pregnancies as we create a birth plan.

Creating a birth plan or developing specific expectations about breastfeeding leaves you with the potential to be greatly disappointed if the reality of the experience does not meet up with the expectation of the experience. I'm all for knowing what you would *like* to have happen during labour and delivery. For example, the desire to be free to walk around or use a birth ball during contractions is fabulous and can be very helpful. But how will you handle your experience if you are told your baby is in distress and you must stay in bed and be constantly monitored? What happens if the messages of society interfere with your plans for birth and cause you to fall victim to the medicalized vision of childbirth? Will you discard all your hopes and plans allowing your doctor to take over the process? And once your baby is born, what will you do if your nurse tells you your baby's blood sugar is low? Will you allow the nurse to begin making choices that will affect your breastfeeding relationship with your child? Will you choose society's medicalized view, believing that formula is the only recourse possible? While plans for how you would like things to happen are well and good, knowing how you will react when things don't go as planned is all the more important.

Being knowledgeable about the birth and breastfeeding experience you would like is recommended. Being knowledgeable about how to *get* the birth and breastfeeding experience you would like is absolutely necessary. Heather had big expectations when it came to breastfeeding, but faced with a difficult labour and a demanding nurse, she found it difficult to follow through with what was necessary. She explains, "My intentions were grand but my will was shattered." When faced with the reality of your experience, even the best-laid plans may prove difficult in the execution. For this reason, it is important to spend time educating yourself, building your positive support system, and considering what you'll do if your expectations are not met. Recognizing the impact of society's many messages about breastfeeding and childbirth is also critical. When faced with difficulties, it is important to make choices that will lessen the impact on breastfeeding initiation.

Our expectations can be dangerous if we aren't able to adapt to an experience that doesn't fit within them, but society's impact and the normalization of formula have created expectations within many new mothers that are more far-reaching and detrimental than many realize. The amount of milk thought to be required by a newborn, for example, is largely skewed by a tacit acceptance of formula feeding as the norm. Many new mothers worry that they don't have enough milk in the early hours and days after their baby is born and often decide—either due to their own worries or the pressure from those around them—to supplement with formula, just until their milk "comes in". Seeing a baby being given a full bottle of formula and then believing that large quantities of milk are normal for a newborn is just one example of how insidious these social messages are and why educating ourselves is so crucial.

Newborns, in fact, require very little milk in the early hours and days following delivery. In fact, nature has created the perfect system to allow babies to slowly initiate their digestive system and gradually increase the amount of milk they ingest. Upon birth, a mother has a significant quantity of colostrum available for the newborn. Breastfeeding soon after delivery ensures a baby receives this colostrum, gives the baby a good dose of immune properties to protect them from the dangers of this new world, and helps initiate the bonding process between mom and baby. Colostrum also acts as a gentle laxative which encourages the removal of meconium present in the baby's intestinal tract.

Frequent nursing during the first hours of life also helps to regulate a mother's milk supply. Milk supply at four and five months post-partum is partially set in the early days following delivery and is strengthened through frequent breast stimulation. As a baby and mom perfect the latch, the breast is still quite soft allowing for easier latching. As the milk supply increases, the baby is ready to take more milk and the need for milk increases. A mother's supply slowly increases after delivery, matching the baby's needs. The baby's stomach size corresponds with the amount of milk available to it. At birth, a baby's stomach is about the size of a small marble, 5-7 millilitres. At three days of age, the stomach has grown to around the size of a larger shooter marble, 0.75- 1 ounce. And by seven days of age, the stomach has reached a capacity of about the size of a ping-pong ball, 1.5-2 ounces.[1] At this size, the baby is feeding quite often ensuring milk is removed frequently and completely which in turn ensures the initiation and continuation of a strong milk supply.

When our expectations of breastfeeding are skewed, or when formula feeding norms are applied to breastfeeding, the impact is often negative. Just one bottle of formula to "top off" the baby can lead to a quick decline in breastfeeding. For this reason, it is not enough to simply intend to breastfeed or want to breastfeed. That desire and intention must be coupled with an understanding of what is normal for breastfeeding, how formula feeding has invaded our society's understanding of what normal newborn feeding looks like, and how you will react in situations that vary from what you hoped would happen—situations that have the potential to affect your end goal: breastfeeding your new baby.

Letting Go of Expectations

When my son was born nine weeks premature, I quickly realized that many of the expectations I had about pregnancy, childbirth, and breastfeeding were not going to be met. We, of course, all have expectations, but the failure to meet expectations or have them come to fruition can leave us with a difficult challenge to overcome. Couple this fact with the emotional aspects of breast-

feeding, and it is apparent that the failure to achieve the expectations of breastfeeding can be overwhelming and create a great
deal of anxiety, anger, hurt, grief, guilt, and sorrow. It is for this
reason that I suggest high expectations and a lack of education
are a dangerous combination.

I'm certainly not suggesting that expectations and plans
should not be part of the preparations for childbirth, but when
we focus too much on the planning and do not spend a significant amount of time filling in the gaps in our knowledge and
preparing ourselves for the possible bumps along the way, the
risk of not meeting our expectations is much greater. Consider,
for example, the amount of time spent learning about and
preparing for breastfeeding compared to time spent learning
about and preparing for childbirth. It is important to educate
yourself about both experiences, yet childbirth is something that
will happen one way or the other; your baby will not remain in
your womb indefinitely. (Although at times it might seem like a
possibility!) However, breastfeeding is not a given. There are
many alternatives to breastfeeding that are common in our
society and numerous potential interferences that can lead away
from a successful breastfeeding relationship. And yet, breastfeeding is, by most expectant mothers, given only a small portion
of time and attention in the months leading up to the baby's
arrival.

Pre-natal classes provide equally insufficient time to truly
educate mothers about normal breastfeeding as they often only
set–aside, out of eight or ten hours of classes, a couple of hours
for breastfeeding, if that. When preparation for breastfeeding is
so insignificant, is it any wonder that we as expectant mothers
have high expectations and yet little understanding about
breastfeeding? Is it any wonder that we go into it completely
unprepared for both what is normal as well as what needs to be
avoided in order to steer clear of common problems? While

having expectations is normal, it is important to let go of those expectations to a certain extent and instead focus on education and preparation for the experience that you will have, allowing yourself to have sufficient knowledge to make decisions that will provide you with the best experience possible. While you can't always choose what will happen to you, you can choose how you react and what you will do with the experience given to you. Unlike expectations, which are fairly slow to change and adapt, *preparation for the experience* will give you the power to shape what happens to you and give you control of your situation.

Reframing the Experience

The difference between *expectations* and *preparation for an experience* may be a subtle one, but it is, I believe, a very important difference. Expectations are set. They don't change. You expect to have a labour without pain control. This is your plan. But when you are faced with a grueling back labour that is painful beyond your wildest imaginings, to then ask for pain control is failing to meet your expectation. However, educating and preparing yourself for how you will deal with pain during labour as opposed to planning *not* to have pain control medications, allows you to make choices given the experience in which you find yourself.

You give yourself the opportunity to weigh your options: is the pain so severe you wish to have an epidural or would a TENS (Transcutaneous Electrical Nerve Stimulation) machine perhaps be a good first option? If you have an epidural, how might that impact the progress of the labour and potentially breastfeeding? What can you do to limit these effects? Having the knowledge behind you, and making decisions based on this knowledge, places you in control, provides you with the knowledge necessary to limit any negative impacts and allows you to put a plan in place in order to achieve your overall objectives.

This may seem rather similar to creating a birth plan and having certain expectations about how childbirth and breastfeeding will happen, but there is one major difference: you have control and are in control. Through education and knowledge, we as women can make choices that are based not on the advice of a doctor, but on facts and research. Your doctor is there to advise you based on his or her knowledge, but your doctor's goals may not be the same as yours. While your doctor's goal is to arrive at the end with a healthy baby and mom, for doctors the process is not always of the foremost importance and how the process might affect activities such as breastfeeding once a baby is born is not always considered. And as we will see in a later chapter, the process is most definitely a continuum. What happens during childbirth can, without a doubt, have a major impact on breastfeeding.

For many women who have struggled with breastfeeding, the feeling of loss can be overwhelming. This sense of loss is often due to the loss of the expectation of breastfeeding—something that was expected that has not been achieved. When we reframe our thinking with regards to our expectations, and instead focus on our reactions to the experience and giving ourselves the tools to make informed choices when faced with an experience other than what we might expect, we can take control of our experience and choose to define our own success based on what is important to us and what is possible given the experience we have.

~~~

The Unplanned Pregnancy

Well the pregnancy itself was planned, but the course of the pregnancy most certainly was not. From the moment the home pregnancy test read positive, I began making plans for my pregnancy. I began to dream of the wonderful moments I would experience over the next forty weeks: the ultrasound, hearing the heartbeat, the first kick, the first time my husband would feel the baby move, the joy of finding out if it was a boy or girl, endless hours poring over baby name books, my last day of work before my maternity leave, the baby shower, the anticipation of those last few weeks before giving birth, the excitement of finally going into labour and knowing that soon I would meet my precious baby.

Being the type of person who loves to be prepared, I spent my spare time reading books about pregnancy, labour and delivery, breastfeeding, and parenthood. I was going to be ready for what lay ahead of me. I carefully considered my options and finely tuned my birth plan so that everyone involved would know my wishes. My expectations began to develop; I had clear ideas of what my pregnancy and delivery would be like.

My pregnancy proceeded problem-free (once I overcame the awe-inspiring morning sickness in the first trimester). At eighteen weeks, I saw my baby for the first time with the ultrasound and found out we were having a boy. More fodder for my planning. I was now able to concentrate on names for boys and focus my shopping on boys' clothing. The nursery plans also abandoned any hope of pink or frilly and took on a decidedly masculine flavour. The anticipation continued to build.

The monthly doctor's visits were really rather uneventful: weight gain good, fundal height right on target, blood pressure normal. Finally at around twenty-eight weeks, my family doctor referred me to an obstetrician. The first visit with the obstetrician was as uneventful as my family doctor visits had been, and it was decided that I would continue to see my family doctor in between visits to the obstetrician. It was my first pregnancy and not knowing what to expect, I enjoyed each day as it came.

So at thirty weeks along in my pregnancy, with everything going exceptionally well, off I went to a regular appointment with my family doctor. From past visits, I knew his scale was a couple of pounds over what my home scale measured, but when I weighed eight pounds more than I had the previous day at home, I began to wonder. He also noted that my blood pressure was a little higher than usual, but still within normal range. I continued to wonder. Then two days later, when my ankles disappeared and tree trunks took their place, I rushed to the local pharmacy to take my blood pressure—165/93! The next morning I was in my doctor's office.

Within three hours of my visit to my doctor, I was being admitted to the hospital with severe preeclampsia. And within three days of being admitted into the hospital, I was being induced. Suddenly, I was thrust into an early end to my pregnancy and a labour for which I was not prepared, one that did not follow my expectations, and one that went beyond anything I had even considered. While I had planned for a labour with as few interventions as possible, here I was have everything I had been sure I did not want now being forced upon me: IV, pitocin, constant monitoring, bed confinement, membranes ruptured. No longer did it seem like I had a choice. Instead, everything was focused on ensuring my baby was delivered safely.

Of course this too was my primary goal, especially when facing the long road that must be traveled when your baby is born prematurely. At thirty-one weeks, there were still many possible complications and our focus was on reducing any possible risks and having a healthy baby. And after a very short labour and quick delivery, our son was born weighing three pounds two ounces and breathing on his own. We were blessed.

It was after the delivery and once I was taken to the mother-baby unit, without my baby, that I started to feel the loss of my pregnancy—the pregnancy I had expected. I began to mourn the loss of my last two months of pregnancy. This was to be the time I was to revel in the anticipation of meeting my son. The time when I would be given a baby shower. The time when I would be doted on as the expectant mother. But all of these expectations were lost.

Once my baby boy arrived, he remained in the NICU for five weeks and the expectations continued to dissolve. Leaving the hospital a few days after delivery without my baby was extremely difficult. Having to return to the hospital every day to visit my baby was a cycle of exhaustion and worry. Breastfeeding suddenly became far more of a challenge than I had ever anticipated, and unexpectedly, I was attached to a breast pump for what seemed like the majority of the day, pumping every two hours. Nothing went as I had planned.

Looking back on that experience from the distance of time, I recognize the strength, knowledge, and lessons my "unexpected" pregnancy and labour brought me. It seems like such a cliché to say the only thing that matters is a healthy baby—but this is the truth! Perhaps living in the moment brings us far greater strength than we could ever anticipate. Expending energy on how we would *like* things to happen removes us from the opportunity to simply *be* there when it does.

The birth of a baby, especially your own, is the greatest time of joy you will ever experience in life. It is the time when all your hopes and dreams take form and are shared with the world. The time when expectations matter very little and reality is present in its simplest, truest form. The moment when a new life ventures into this world for the first time and seeks out your face because you are its mother.

Breastfeeding, Take Two

An Experience by Any Other Name...

"I always based my expectations on her experiences and just assumed I would nurse the same amount."

Caroline, mom of four

B efore moving on to the second section of this book, the section devoted to more specific actions and ideas to help achieve a positive breastfeeding outcome, it is important to spend a bit of time discussing the language surrounding breastfeeding and how, by changing the language and our discussions about breastfeeding, we can also move towards changing our outcomes.

Breastfeeding as Normal

Earlier in the book we discussed the popular and successful slogan "breast is best" that has been promoted over the past decade or so to encourage women to breastfeed. While at its heart this slogan has been intended to encourage breastfeeding and highlight that breastfeeding has benefit over formula, it has ultimately served to create a view of breastfeeding as an excellent choice but it maintains formula feeding as the central, and perhaps even normal, method of infant feeding.

Stating that breastfeeding is "best" by default suggests that the alternative is good. Formula, according to the "breast is best" slogan, must be a good alternative, with breastfeeding of course being an even better choice. By positioning one option as the best, it has added to the guilt women feel as a result of their choice to feed infant formula or their inability to breastfeed. It doesn't take into account the lack of information or support available to women or the pressures placed on new mothers from society and big business. Breastfeeding is best, and if you are a good mother, you do what is best, right?

It doesn't take much consideration to recognize how "breast is best" might actually undermine the efforts of breastfeeding moms. We all want to do what is best for our children, and we as mothers make choices that, we hope, are in the best interests of our children. Breastfeeding is best, but when a baby won't latch or your nipples are so painful you simply can't continue nursing, and there is nowhere to turn for accurate advice and support, we are at least consoled by the fact that while breastfeeding is best, formula is still good.

And it is good. Do not misunderstand my intentions here. Formula most definitely has its place. Using it is a lifesaving measure and we are fortunate to live in a time and a society that allows us to have access to a safe, alternative method for feeding our infants (although if milk banks were given the support and funding they deserve, less formula would be required). Yet it is important to understand how the dialogue of our society affects our own internal dialogue and the way we view our parenting experiences.

There is a growing movement in the lactation community that recognizes the "breast is best" campaign has not caused the rise in breastfeeding rates that was hoped for. Everyone knows the slogan, intentions to breastfeed are high, and yet breastfeeding rates are dismally low. Where have we gone wrong? If breast-feeding is best, why isn't everyone breastfeeding?

As alluded to earlier in the book, we have a society that pro-claims support for breastfeeding and yet gives little real support. As new moms, we are told it is important and something we should do if we want the "best" for our babies; however, we are given few resources to help ensure success. Breastfeeding is heralded as the ultimate in infant nutrition, and yet baby bottles are used as the symbol of babies everywhere and every baby doll comes with its own baby bottle. Exclusive breastfeeding is recommended for the first six months of a baby's life with continued breastfeeding up to two years of age and beyond, and yet in the United States a mother is lucky to get a few weeks off of work after the arrival of her baby. We have an extreme divide between what the "breast is best" slogan suggests and what our society is willing to support. What is needed is a change of focus and a reframing of the entire issue.

That reframing needs to start with how *we* view — and dis-cuss — breastfeeding. If we look at it as the best option, then, as mentioned above, this means that other options are good. Instead, if we change our view and begin to see breastfeeding as "normal" we also begin to view it in its rightful biological perspective and, when seen in this way, we can make choices and support breastfeeding on a continuum of normal — giving us a higher likelihood of success.

Breastfeeding is biologically normal. As discussed in an ear-lier chapter, we are biological creatures and as mammals we are intended to feed our infants at our breast. This is just the way it is and we cannot avoid this truth. As a biologically normal act, it is ruled by biological processes and events. Instead of simply calling it "best" but not being given any support or information to help achieve successful breastfeeding, viewing and discussing breastfeeding as "normal" provides us with a large amount of knowledge based on biology and normal biological processes. No longer is breastfeeding about rules and gadgets, now it can be about your body and your baby and the biological processes at work. Once you understand the processes, and things that might interfere with them, you have far more knowledge at your disposal to make breastfeeding work for you.

Making this shift in thinking can be challenging. We have been raised in a world where our biology is considered embarrassing, something to be ignored or even hidden as much as possible—we are enlightened creatures after all. Modern society does not like to think of humans as biological beings as though being so is somehow a negative condition. When we distance ourselves from our biological selves it creates a division between what our biological selves expect and what our society expects. During motherhood, we as women are closest to our biological selves. We have biological drives to mother and to nurture and nourish our children. Listening to our inner voice and following our maternal instincts can be challenging given the distractions of our society, but when we strive to listen it becomes easier to parent. When we are not fighting our biological needs with regards to breastfeeding, breastfeeding too happens more easily.

This is not to say that a simple shift in thinking, and calling breastfeeding biologically normal instead of best, is going to make all the difference and that no one who thinks of breastfeeding in this way will ever have difficulties breastfeeding again. That would just be silly. It will help though and can also assist you in accessing information and support that is conducive to success instead of counterproductive to it since you can focus only on information that views breastfeeding as biologically normal, but difficulties will still arise. And when they do, it's important to try and view the challenges as opportunities and lessons. These lessons are often the most valuable ones we learn in life.

Is it really failure?

The beginning of this book mentions the discomfort I have surrounding the word "failure" when it comes to breastfeeding. Instead of fighting the word, I've chosen to embrace it and use it when necessary within this book to describe the inability to initiate or maintain a breastfeeding relationship. But really, I'm not sure "failure" is the best word to describe the situation. I do know that it is rarely a failure on the part of the mother and never a failure on the part of the baby when breastfeeding does not work out.

If breastfeeding is viewed as the *normal* process instead of the *best* choice, we might see breastfeeding failure as a deviation from that normal process. There are many things that can cause this type of deviation: birth interventions, scheduling feedings, early bottle use, mother and baby separation. Often things that can derail the natural process are even recommended to us by doctors and nurses (such as giving formula in the hospital so mom can get some rest) or encouraged by family and friends (who very often did not breastfeed their own children). It can be easy to fall off the path that our biology expects us to follow. This can't be seen as a failure but instead a situation where we have been misled or have gone astray.

Breastfeeding failure might also be viewed as a lack of information. Often, even though we search for information, we do not find the information we need. The market is flooded with books about childbirth and breastfeeding. Some are great and some aren't. How do you as a new mom know the difference? How is it your failure when you tried to access information, read the books, took the classes, and were given information that was inconsistent, inaccurate, outdated, or against our biological nature? This isn't your failure. When you do the best you can with the information you have, there is no blame to be placed on you. While you might still feel that you failed at breastfeeding, place the blame where it belongs. If, knowing breastfeeding was best for your baby, you just gave up without really trying or making any effort to make it work, then maybe it is yours to bear. But most women I know honestly try everything at their disposal and simply cannot access the information they need or the support they deserve.

Failure to find the support you need to make breastfeeding work is also common. Again, when you have sought support and have been unable to find what you need, this isn't your failure. This failure lands squarely on society's shoulders. Our "breast is best" society has created a generation of doctors who believe that while breast may be best, formula is okay too. We tell women they should breastfeed, all the while closing down breastfeeding clinics or not opening them in the first place. You may be fortunate to have family and friends surrounding you who are supportive, and yet when you walk out your front door you walk into a world that asks women to nurse their babies in the bathroom while bare breasts are shown on television and in the movies.

Breastfeeding failure. Yes, we have failed at breastfeeding. But more often than not, the failure is not the failure of the mother or the baby. Our society has failed us. This is not to say that sometimes new mothers couldn't have done more or should not have made different choices. Sure, we all sometimes make mistakes. Perhaps breastfeeding wasn't really important to the mother or she wasn't really comfortable with it. That's okay. While breastfeeding is biologically normal and expected, we do live in a world that tries hard to ignore our biological natures.

Embrace where you are; recognize why you feel this way; decide whether it's something you truly wish to change. If you don't want to breastfeed, don't. But make that decision from a place of knowledge and power. Understand the truths about breastfeeding and the reasons for your own views and opinions.

Take control of your own choice instead of allowing marketing and society's views to make your choices for you.

Defining Your Own Success

If you are reading this book, you have likely had a breastfeeding experience that was less than you expected it to be. Maybe it never really started or perhaps it ended much earlier than you had hoped it would end. While we don't necessarily choose the experiences we are given, we can change how we view them and how we react to them. Being able to view and talk about difficulties and failure in a different way can help to make your experience one that is ultimately positive.

Expectations often leave us feeling as though it is an all or nothing proposition. If your expectation is that you will breastfeed, at what point will you have succeeded? Will you need to breastfeed for four weeks, six months, two years? Does breastfeeding mean no bottles will ever be used or that any formula would be considered a failure? In her essay "Drained" in *Unbuttoned*, Jennifer Restaino clearly focuses on the impact of her expectations saying, "What I saw as my 'failures' as a new mother were just that: all mine...I realized that it had been, always, a battle with my own expectations."[1] When we bring with us expectations for how something will turn out, it is often difficult to make changes midcourse if necessary. Rather than having expectations, moving forward with strong intentions is a better mindset to have.

Giving yourself permission to make decisions, based on the experience you are given, is crucial, as opposed to having expectations for how the experience will turn out. You never know what life will throw at you, and it is important to allow yourself the ability to change mid-flight if necessary. Instead of thinking in terms of expectations, formulate your aspirations.

Learning to change our expectations to aspirations can be challenging, as I learned firsthand.

When my daughter was born, I was completely committed to the idea of babywearing. My plan was to wear my baby in a wrap frequently and keep her close. This was all well and good until my lovely daughter was born and presented herself as what I affectionately refer to as a "motion junkie". She was a lovely, happy baby as long as she was moving. She would sleep like a dream on car rides—until the car stopped at a light. She would happily sleep all day snuggled against my chest in a wrap, but the moment I set her down she was miserable. You can imagine how this affected her ability to sleep at night! I had always said I would never use an infant swing to keep my child busy, and I fought it for awhile, until it was either my sanity or my daughter that was going to have to go! I went out to WalMart and purchased a swing and there she slept every night until she was almost six months old. I wanted her to co-sleep—would have been more than happy to have her with me in bed—but she was miserable laying flat and still. She would kick and thrash all night long, not only keeping herself up, but keeping me up as well.

My daughter's sleeping arrangements were not what I ever expected them to be. It was not what I wanted. But given the reality of our experience, I had to alter my plans and change my idea of what "successful" parenting would look like for me. Success initially would have been co-sleeping and having a happy baby who loved to sleep. Being able to change my definition of success was necessary, and while I didn't get to co-sleep as much as I'd like, my daughter was worn in her wrap frequently and we enjoyed a wonderful closeness in that way. My daughter didn't sleep through the night until she was two years old. From her, I learned that what you want and what you get are often two very different things. Being able to alter your plans to fit your reality is critical.

Being able to alter your vision of success when it comes to breastfeeding is also important. Having a grand, overall goal is fantastic, but also realizing that sometimes alterations need to be made to our plans is important. It is never an all or nothing proposition. Paula Spencer, in her essay "Step One, Try It; Step Two, Whatever Works" in *Unbuttoned*, presents a simple definition of success: "...everybody coming out okay."[2] "Okay" might be different for everyone. But it is important not to get lost in the struggle and lose sight of what is most important to you. The struggle can be overwhelming to some and each woman will have her own limit. Understanding these limits, and realizing the options available to you once you reach this limit, is important.

When it comes to breastfeeding, there are many variations possible: exclusive breastfeeding, supplementing, exclusive pumping, partial breastfeeding and pumping. You likely have an understanding of some of these variations from your first breastfeeding experience. Exclusive breastfeeding should be the first option if possible, but it's not always possible. If you do choose another alternative, it is important to understand how the variation may affect your breastfeeding relationship or your milk supply and ensure you follow good breastfeeding/pumping protocols to limit any negative consequences. One of the most important things to understand when breastfeeding is that your milk supply is of utmost importance. Protect your milk supply at all costs. When you have milk to provide to your baby, you have options. Success for you may mean breastfeeding for six months, expressing for a year, or allowing your child to self-wean at three years of age, but without a good milk supply, your options are greatly limited. Regardless of your definition of success, establish a strong supply and work to maintain it.

In this first section of the book, I have tried to explore what breastfeeding failure is and isn't, some of the reasons why breastfeeding is such an emotional experience, how these emotions play into our ability or inability to breastfeed, how society influences breastfeeding, how guilt affects us when breastfeeding doesn't work out and how what we feel is more accurately called grief, how we might better focus on the experience instead of the expectations surrounding birth and breastfeeding, and the importance of renaming our "failure" and recognizing the many influences that affect our ability to breastfeed.

The next section of the book will delve into more concrete issues affecting breastfeeding. It will provide a basic overview of lactation and the biological processes that are critical to the establishment of a successful breastfeeding relationship, what normal breastfeeding and mothering looks like, how to make plans to succeed at breastfeeding with your next baby, and considers the possibility of it not working out a second time.

~·~·~

Laura's Story

During my pregnancy, I thought breastfeeding was the only rational choice: best for infants, environmentally sound, a wonderful bonding experience between mother and child. My doctor warned me that it wasn't "natural" —she described it as a skill to be learned, like driving a manual transmission—and I committed to learning the skill. I felt mentally prepared, yet conscious that I had a great deal to learn. I had planned to breastfeed until my son weaned himself, although I wanted to introduce a daily bottle of pumped breast milk fairly early, so that my husband could participate in our son's feeding.

My son latched beautifully minutes after birth, my milk came in quickly, and he thrived. But from the beginning, we had enormous difficulty persuading him to sleep: he averaged a total of eight hours' sleep in every twenty-four hour period, and needed to be rocked/shushed/soothed/worn even to achieve this meagre amount of rest. Because my husband and I were so very sleep-deprived, I didn't realize that we were having breastfeeding difficulties until my son was two weeks old. He bit at the breast, thrashed, and actively nursed for sixty to eighty minutes per session. I did constant compressions and dared not relax my C-hold. Nursing was a tense, two-handed operation during which I could neither relax nor multi-task, and I dreaded each upcoming feed. He nursed every two hours around the clock (twelve sessions in twenty-four hours), so by the end of two weeks I was too sore to get dressed. I didn't leave the house (except for medical appointments) because it was too painful to wear a bra and shirt. I called my doula, who suggested that I may have an overactive let-down and suggested I nurse reclined. This did not help. She then suggested I see a lactation consultant.

The first LC checked my son's latch (pronounced it "A-1") and instructed me, when he bit, to take him off the breast, calm him, and put him back on. This did nothing to help, especially since my son only calmed when put back on the breast.

I then saw my doctor (a qualified LC), who checked my son's latch and, after some questions, prescribed medications for acid reflux. We saw no results from these at the end of two more weeks.

I saw an LC for the third time, who checked my son's latch (still "first class!") and refused to believe that my son was nursing for the durations I told her. She told me that I must be falling asleep and losing track of the time. When I said that I was much too tense to have a conversation, let alone fall asleep, she told me that my tension was inhibiting his ability to nurse and that if I just relaxed, he would stop biting.

I asked each of these experts if it was possible that I simply didn't have enough milk. Their response each time was that I clearly had enough, because my son was gaining weight appropriately.

At the two-month mark, my son was still biting (at least once per nursing session), still nursing twelve times in twenty-four hours, and for 45-80 minutes per session. He still only slept when worn in a carrier—and I was falling apart. I bought a dual electric pump, ate oatmeal, took fenugreek seeds by the tablespoonful, and tried exclusively pumping (EP). My goal was to do this until he was six months old. This was equally disastrous, because it meant that it doubled our feeding time. It took me forty-five minutes to pump a 4-5 oz. bottle of milk; it took my husband that long to persuade our son to drink it. Between feeding, diaper changes, and rocking our son to sleep, we had thirty minutes of "free time" in each twenty-four hour period. After a month, we packed it in. We transitioned from breast milk to formula over a three-week period and by four months of age, our son was fully formula-fed. We were still miserable, but less so than before.

It took me several weeks truly to understand that there are two people in a breastfeeding relationship. No matter how much the mother desires success, how skilled she becomes, and how diligent she is, that this is only half the issue. At two years of age, my son is still a biter: sippy cups, straws, drinking spouts—he has never stopped clamping down. He's still a slow eater, spinning out meals for thirty-five to forty minutes when his peers are done in ten to fifteen. He's still "thrashy"—kicking his feet constantly as he sits in his high chair, running circles around dogs in the park. But he's happy and bright and thriving. Twelve months of formula didn't make him fat or stupid or a picky eater.

If I had the chance to do this again, I would get help earlier; be much more assertive with the LCs and my doctor, rejecting especially the insinuations that I was either neurotic, a liar, or a half-wit (I was too tired and too worried about my son to defend myself at the time); push harder about the possibility of not having enough milk; and accept that I can't let down for a pump. Had we been less sleep-deprived, I would have made an appointment with Dr. Jack Newman. At the time, however, a trip to the grocery store had to be planned like a military mission. There was no way we could have driven to Toronto.

This experience had both immediate and long-term effects. At the time, I was devastated and felt, very starkly, that I had failed my son. I was angry and defensive and was ashamed to be seen giving him a bottle. I was furious, too, that I couldn't pump enough milk to nourish him exclusively on breast milk. I avoided conversations about nursing at all costs.

As for the long-term effects, one unexpected benefit to not having been able to breastfeed is that my husband was highly involved in our son's early feeding. It's helped us to share our parenting as equally as possible, and I see this in my son's incredibly strong attachment to his father. When our son is injured, he runs not necessarily to me, but to whomever's closer—something I credit, in part, to the bottle I fought so hard against.

I think breastfeeding is presented in an overly simplistic, idealized light—as though it's as simple as "choosing" to breastfeed and "hanging in there through the initial discomfort". I'm still frustrated that three lactation consultants, using the La Leche League manual, were unable to help us. If we have another baby I will make every effort to breastfeed, but my hopes for success will be tempered by this experience. I'll ask for help earlier but if it is still excruciatingly difficult for no clear reason, I will give myself permission to stop and focus on the myriad things I *can* do for my child.

Section Two

Taking Control of the Experience

Let's Get Back to Basics

"The amount of advice and counseling one could get, the sheer number of contraptions one could invest in, the full gamut of books that were available for sale came at me with a dizzying pace leaving me utterly bewildered."

Michelle, mom of one

I n an age in which information is quickly disseminated and easily accessed, both the lack of information and indeed the misinformation about breastfeeding are shocking. Much of the information readily available is superficial at best, and all too often breastfeeding information is based on formula feeding as the norm. But in order to take back control of breastfeeding's role in our culture, it is important to begin accessing and sharing information that is based on a view of breastfeeding as the biologically normal method of infant feeding. Understanding the biological realities of lactation and the normal behaviour of a newborn, and how that behaviour impacts the initiation of lactation and milk supply, are important to getting off to a good start. When we approach breastfeeding from a bottle-feeding perspective, we are interfering with the processes that help to ensure successful breastfeeding. Cynthia Good Mojab explains, "When breastfeeding knowledge has been lost in individual families and entire societies, the techniques that are appropriate for formula feeding—such as scheduled, infrequent, time-

153

limited, and measured feedings—are applied to breastfeeding."[1] Applying these formula feeding techniques to breastfeeding greatly affects the outcomes for breastfeeding. There are never any guarantees, but having accurate information will go a long way to getting you where you want to be. And if problems do arise, having accurate information based on breastfeeding as the biologically normal feeding method will help you make decisions that increase the chances of a successful outcome.

What follows is information that you may never have been given, or the impact of which on breastfeeding you may not fully have realized. The following pages will examine the process of lactation; the continuum of pregnancy, birth, and breastfeeding; the importance of skin-to-skin time with baby; the possible impact of birth interventions; and what normal mothering looks like from a biological perspective.

Critical Factors in Milk Production

An understanding of the process of lactation is important for all mothers. Understanding how lactation is initiated and regulated can help you establish a strong milk supply, maintain that supply, make decisions that reduce any potential impact to the breastfeeding relationship, and understand how newborn behaviour serves to ensure a good breastfeeding outcome.

Stages of Lactation

Lactogenesis I begins during pregnancy. The mammary glands change from inactive to active preparing for lactation. About half-way through pregnancy, the breasts will begin to produce colostrum. You may or may not experience leaking at this time. Breasts usually enlarge, veins become darker, the areolas enlarge and darken, and the nipples become more erect.

Lactogenesis II begins following the detachment of the placenta. This stage of lactation is triggered by a sharp decline of progesterone following the detachment and subsequent delivery of the placenta. Any retained placenta can greatly affect a mother's ability to establish a full milk supply.

Colostrum is present at birth and is all a baby requires until milk production increases. Colostrum is high in antibodies and protein, has a laxative effect which assists the baby in removing meconium from its system, and coats the gut providing protection from potential pathogens. It's important to realize that a baby's environment is sterile until birth. Once born, a baby is suddenly exposed to a host of dangers. Nature has provided the initial dose of colostrum as an "inoculation" against these many dangers. Since the mother has already been exposed to these dangers in the environment, her colostrum will provide antibodies against these elements specific to her environment.

Formula provided during this time (even just once) changes the normal flora of the gut and it can take days for it to return to normal. Marsha Walker has created a fantastic handout that reviews the research as it relates to the risks of feeding formula to breastfed babies.[2] The gut flora of a breastfed baby is significantly different from that of a formula-fed baby. If we believe that breastfeeding is normal, then we must also believe that this difference is significant and strive to maintain a normal balance in our baby's system.

Milk production slowly increases over the first few days postpartum. It usually takes two to five days for milk volumes to increase, but it can take longer depending on certain factors such as certain birth interventions or medical conditions. First-time mothers will see an increase later than mothers with previous children.

Milk will slowly transition from colostrum to mature milk. Mature milk will usually have a bluish colour but can vary in colour due to the mother's diet. Breast milk usually looks quite thin and watery and will separate with a thick creamy layer on top if expressed and left to sit. For a breastfeeding mother, the colour and appearance of breast milk really isn't too much of a concern.

It is important to realize that lactogenesis II will happen regardless of whether a woman is choosing to nurse her baby, express her breast milk, or formula feed her child since lactogenesis II is a result of hormonal factors.

The Hormones Involved

Prolactin

Prolactin is the hormone responsible for triggering milk production. It is also referred to as a "mothering hormone" because it creates mothering responses. Prolactin levels rise sharply following delivery and fall substantially over the first twenty-four to thirty-six hours post-partum. Prolactin is produced by the anterior pituitary gland and causes a decrease in estrogen levels. Levels of this hormone vary throughout the day with the highest levels at night; hence the importance of breastfeeding around the clock and during the night. Most newborns want to nurse around the clock, and while this may be tiring or inconvenient, it really is the best way to make use of these high prolactin levels and initiate a strong supply. Once lactation is established, prolactin takes on only a permissive role as opposed to a regulatory role meaning that it no longer drives production but its presence simply allows milk production to continue.

Oxytocin

Oxytocin is vital during both the birthing process (contractions) and lactation (milk ejection reflex). It is also a "loving hormone" assisting in creating affection and social bonds with others. Oxytocin can help to create a relaxed, calm, and euphoric feeling which both the mother and the baby experience. Oxytocin is important to the bonding of mother and baby and, in the presence of prolactin and its influence on mothering responses, oxytocin helps to create a strong bond between mom and baby. Oxytocin levels in the brain soar immediately after delivery—one reason why immediate and uninterrupted one-on-one time following a baby's birth is so important.

Endocrine and Autocrine Control

Endocrine control refers to the hormonally driven stage of lactation—Lactogenesis II—which will happen regardless of whether a baby is nursing or not (with rare exceptions such as Sheehan's Syndrome or physiological conditions such as hypoplasia) and lasts for a few weeks after a baby is born. During this time, lactation is established and supply is set. Milk production will vary depending on the amount of stimulation to the breasts, nipples, and areolas, and the frequency of stimulation. This is an amazing aspect of nature since the variation in frequency helps a mother regulate her milk supply depending on the number of babies she has. So milk supply will be different for the mother of a single baby as opposed to the mother of twins. But this also means that limiting a newborn's access to the breast, scheduling feedings, or using formula to supplement even just once in a while, can affect milk supply in both the short-term and the long-term. And for this reason, it is vitally important that breastfeeding happens frequently.

Autocrine (local) control is also referred to as lactogenesis III and is the maintenance stage of lactation. This relies on the principle of supply and demand, and it is both interesting and important to know that milk synthesis is controlled at the breast.

Two Key Processes Controlling Milk Production

Milk removal is the primary control mechanism for milk supply. In other words, milk removed from the breast initiates more production of milk in the breast. As the scientific community continues to research lactation, the understanding of milk production continues to develop. One of the most important things to understand about lactation and milk production is this: Milk production slows as the breast fills!

Far too often I read or hear women telling other women that perhaps they are not waiting long enough for their breasts to "fill up" again in between feedings and that this is why they don't have enough milk. This well-meaning advice is simply wrong and goes against everything science teaches us about the process of lactation. If you want to produce enough milk you must nurse your baby frequently and allow your baby to remove as much milk as possible from the breast. Milk left sitting in the breast slows production. There are two reasons for this:

> 1.) A mother's milk contains a protein called Feedback Inhibitor of Lactation (FIL). As the breast fills naturally more FIL is present and production will begin to slow. Think of this process as a grocery conveyor belt. As you put groceries onto the belt, you have less and less room to add more and eventually you must stop adding anything because you have run out of room. In order to allow more groceries to be added—or breast milk to be produced— you must remove some of the groceries—or milk. Anyone who has ever suffered from engorgement will appreciate this little protein. It is important to have some limits on the production or else engorgement, plugged ducts, and mastitis would be far more prevalent than they already are.

2.) When the alveoli (small sacs that contain milk-producing cells) are full of milk, their walls expand and the shape of the prolactin receptors change. (You'll remember that prolactin is the hormone that both initiates lactation and allows lactation to continue.) This prevents prolactin from entering at these sites and, as a result, slows milk production. As the alveoli empty, the receptors return to their normal shape allowing prolactin to enter again and milk production to increase.

These two processes are key to understanding milk production. Both frequency and efficiency of milk removal are primary in the initiation and continuation of production. Anything that interferes with these two aspects has the potential to interfere with or harm the breastfeeding relationship.[3]

The Prolactin Receptor Theory

The prolactin receptor theory is another important concept in lactation and has important implications for all breastfeeding moms. The basic idea of the prolactin receptor theory is that milk production is "set" during the first few days and weeks postpartum. Frequent stimulation increases the number of prolactin receptors in the breast allowing the body to utilize prolactin more effectively. This sets the milk production for the rest of the lactation period. Newborns naturally feed for short periods but feed very frequently. This encourages the increase of prolactin receptors and the establishment of a strong milk supply. For mothers who are using a breast pump to initiate their milk supply, it is vitally important to understand the prolactin receptor theory and ensure a pumping schedule that provides frequent stimulation and removal of milk.

The most important aspect of the prolactin receptor theory that all new mothers need to understand is that the newborn's desire to seemingly breastfeed all the time is biology's way of ensuring the mother's milk supply is ample five months or more down the road. Even though it may seem that there is no milk in the breast and that your baby is getting "nothing" a newborn who is nursing frequently is getting exactly what is needed and ensuring that will continue as he or she grows and develops. Hospital practices that separate mom and baby, birth interventions that prevent a baby from nursing within the first hour following delivery, or early bottle supplementation all impact this natural process and interfere with the normal development of prolactin receptors that are critical to long-term breastfeeding.

Storage Capacity and Milk Production

Storage capacity is the amount of milk the breast can hold between nursing or pumping sessions. Storage capacity is not directly related to the size of the breast and can differ between breasts. Storage capacity of the breast impacts the rate of milk production. A large storage capacity will allow milk production to continue for a greater length of time before slowing since the receptors will not "stretch" until full. Think of this concept as a cup: you can drink a large amount of water throughout the day using any size of cup. If you use a small cup you will simply have to refill more often.[4] This is not an indication that a woman with a larger storage capacity can produce more milk, only that a woman with a smaller storage capacity will need to nurse, or pump, more frequently.

It is important to recognize that your storage capacity may affect your baby's feeding pattern. Mothers who have a smaller storage capacity will likely have babies that nurse more frequently. This is important for both the mom's milk supply and for the baby's sufficient intake. Mothers who have a larger storage capacity may have babies who go a little longer between nursing sessions, depending on the amount of milk a baby wants when nursing, but a larger storage capacity will also more than likely affect the pattern of nursing. A baby whose mother has a large storage capacity will more likely feed from only one breast when nursing as opposed to nursing from both breasts during each feeding. All of this really points to the need to listen to our babies and follow their leads. As a mom we are unlikely to truly know if we have a small or large storage capacity, but our babies are working on instinct and are capable of sending cues to let us know that they need more food.

Fat Content

The concept of foremilk and hindmilk is a rather outdated one. Research has shown that fat is released into milk as the breast empties.[5] A baby fed from a full breast will have an increasing amount of fat as the breast empties and a baby fed from a less full breast will have a more consistent level of fat throughout the feed. Likewise, milk that is pumped from a full breast will have an increasing amount of fat as the breast empties. If you express your milk you will notice milk that is first expressed is thinner and more watery, and milk that is expressed from a breast that is not exceedingly full will have a fairly consistent level of fat throughout the pumping session.

A baby's intake, and *not* the amount of fat in breast milk, is the *only* thing that has been connected to infant growth. As long as you are nursing frequently, emptying the breasts as complete-ly as possible during each nursing session, and allowing your baby to determine how often and how long nursing sessions last, you really do not need to be worrying about the fat content of your breast milk. Having said that, it is important to realize that the type of fat in your breast milk is largely influenced by the type of fat in your diet. So do avoid the nasty trans-fats and opt for healthier unsaturated fats and omega fats. If you try to eat a healthy diet, the composition of your milk shouldn't be a concern for you.

Baby Knows Best

Babies have an amazing and innate ability to know what they need. Whether it is human contact, a soothing voice, or a quiet room, once a baby gets what he or she needs, contentment usually follows. The same is true for their feeding. It can be difficult to trust our babies, but while we as mothers would like to be the experts on our children, even as young infants, they do tend to understand what they need perhaps better than we understand what they need. This is a direct result of their understanding of the world as biological creatures instead of as social creatures. Babies know when they need to eat and they know how much they need to eat. We are not born knowing how to overeat or preferring to eat chocolate over healthier options. These things are socialized into us and are a result of our environment and society. For this reason if for no other, it is so important that we learn to trust our babies and allow them some autonomy in their eating.

An interesting story from my own life illustrates this point well. As I've mentioned earlier, my son was born nine weeks premature and because of his small size at birth and his early arrival into the world, he was followed closely through the developmental follow-up program at a local hospital. In the hospital he grew quickly reaching about eight pounds by his due date. While he was a pleasantly chubby baby, he was never big and always weighed in around the twentieth percentile. Once he reached about seven months corrected age, his growth slowed significantly. Concerned, the doctor and dietician from the follow-up program asked me to fortify my expressed milk with formula to boost the caloric content. While not thrilled with the idea (I was, after all, exclusively pumping partly to avoid feeding my son formula), I followed their instructions and began fortifying my milk. And then an amazing thing happened. Almost immediately upon adding the formula to the breast milk, my son reduced his intake. I strongly believe my son innately knew how many calories he needed and adjusted his intake accordingly. My daughter, who was exclusively breastfed, followed exactly the same growth pattern as my son and today both are healthy and normal-weight kids. Trust your baby and follow their lead.

What does this all mean for breastfeeding?

This information is interesting, but what does it all mean when you are actually faced with those sleepless nights, a tiny baby to care for, emotions that are taking you to places you've never been, and feeling as though you've been hit by a truck? This is where nature really shines, for in reality, all the science and biological processes really do not matter as long as we listen to our babies, trust our bodies, and allow our instincts to guide us.

The two things I suggest every mother know are how to determine if her newborn is getting enough milk and how to read her baby's signals that indicate the need to nurse. Throw out all the other "rules" that society gives you and ignore the warnings that picking your baby up when it cries or allowing your baby to fall asleep at the breast will only create bad habits. Think about these things from the biological perspective. Does a mother bear watch the clock to determine how frequently to feed her cubs? Are puppies forced to sleep on their own? Our children are born with needs. This is fact. And these needs are far more complex than simply the need for food and a place to sleep.

Our babies need closeness, body contact, love, movement, interaction, stimulation (and protection from over-stimulation), trust, and a myriad of other things. Meeting our babies' needs will not create dependency; meeting our babies' needs will prepare them to move on to the next stages in their lives without any holes in their development.[6] A number of years ago I heard the statement "meet the need and the need goes away" and it really hit home with me. Not meeting the early needs of our children does not remove those needs. It may train them not to ask us to fill the need, but the need is still there. So when it comes to breastfeeding, your first, and really only, job is to meet the needs of your baby.

Feeding Cues

Babies are fairly subtle when it comes to making their needs known. In order to "hear" their signals, it is important to keep them close. Because frequent breastfeeding is important in establishing milk supply in the hours and days following delivery, it is essential to provide your baby with frequent access to the breast. Sometimes it seems as though your baby is speaking an alien language and you may be concerned that you'll never understand when they need to nurse. In the early days, every time a baby wakes up is a good time to put them to the breast. If a baby is a little fussy, put them to the breast. In other words, offer lots and often. You can never offer too much, but you can certainly offer too little. Frequency of stimulation is important, so even if your baby only nurses briefly, don't worry.

You will eventually figure out your baby's own way of communicating and breastfeeding will fall into a fairly routine pattern after a few weeks, but early on it is important to recognize the normal indicators that a baby needs to nurse. As mentioned above, anytime a baby wakes up is a good time to nurse. But aside from that, reading your baby's early feeding cues helps to prevent your baby from becoming overly upset or hungry. Once a baby is exhibiting late feeding cues, it can be very difficult to get your baby calmed enough to latch and nurse. You never want to try to latch a screaming baby. Instead, bring your baby back to a calm state and then offer the breast. Trying to latch a screaming baby usually just results in a screaming baby.

Early feeding cues include:
- smacking or licking lips
- opening and closing mouth
- sucking on hands, fists, fingers, toys, or clothing

Active feeding cues include:
- rooting, turning towards stimulus on cheek
- trying to position self for feeding
- fidgeting or squirming, hitting you repeatedly on the chest
- fussing

Late feeding cues include:
- moving head frantically from side to side
- crying

Newborn Feeding Patterns

Frequency is the only aspect that will be consistent with a newborn's feeding. There is no schedule to a newborn's feeding pattern, nor should there be. Follow your baby's lead and trust your instincts. Learn about the latch and what a good latch looks like and learn to recognize if your baby is actually drawing milk and actively drinking. If your baby is sleeping for lengthy periods and not nursing or is nursing for excessively long periods, you need to look at whether your baby is nursing effectively. Educating yourself on what to look for will help you determine if and when you need to seek out support and assistance from a lactation consultant.

This book is not intended to be a how-to breastfeeding manual. For that, I highly recommend *Breastfeeding Made Simple* by Nancy Mohrbacher and Kathleen Kendall-Tackett.[7] However, I think the one big question that all new mothers have is whether their baby is getting enough milk. For this reason, I have included information on how to know if your baby is getting enough milk in the appendix of the book.

Effects of Labour Interventions

For some reason, the lists of risks of labour interventions rarely include the significant impact they can have on breastfeeding. Mary Kroeger states that "there is a persistent failure on the part of both obstetrics and paediatrics to disclose to pregnant women the full range of possible side effects of labor pain medications."[8] Many in the medical profession will go so far as to emphatically state that there is no danger to breastfeeding from any intervention that might be used during a woman's labour. However, this stems, I believe, from a lack of awareness of the continuum of pregnancy, childbirth, and breastfeeding. Without seeing these as interconnected aspects of the same process, each is considered as a separate stage and as doctors often acknowledge, their main role in the process of childbirth is to make sure we have a healthy baby and healthy mother at the end.

This, of course, is desired by all involved; however, healthy babies and mothers also have the biological expectation to breastfeed and when interventions impact this natural continuum, they also have the potential to affect the health of mothers and babies and the initiation of breastfeeding.

Birth interventions have significant potential to disrupt breastfeeding. This is not to say interventions will make breastfeeding impossible, but they have the potential to make breastfeeding more difficult and, if there are any other risk factors present including a lack of information or lack of support, interventions can create enormous challenges. From her own experience, IBCLC Judith Gutowski explains, "I rarely see an infant that was born without anaesthesia, without pitocin exposure, without separation from the mother or other trouble-some interventions. The difference in feeding instincts and ability of mother and baby are profound for those who manage to avoid intervention and be born naturally."[9] Knowing that certain interventions can make breastfeeding difficult can help you to be proactive and keep you focused on what you need to do in order to give the breastfeeding relationship the best start possible.

It's important to state here that the following information is not intended to suggest these interventions do not have their place or that they should be wholly avoided. Every medical intervention has the potential to be life-saving in the proper situation; at the same time, every intervention has the potential to be both misused and over-used. As in all other areas discussed in this book, I encourage you to seek out information about birth interventions and become your own advocate when it comes to your maternity care. Always ask for options and alternatives. Arm yourself with information to understand when certain interventions are appropriate and when they are medically unnecessary—yes, some are unnecessary.

In my own experience, I found after a speedy labour and quick delivery of my second child, that even having made it clear to the hospital staff that I wanted my daughter with me immedi-ately after delivery to allow her to nurse for the first time and provide us time to bond, I had to fight with my L & D nurse to give my daughter back to me and not to do a heel prick to test her blood sugar. My daughter had latched on within about twenty minutes of her birth, and we had lain quietly for another forty minutes or so before the nurse returned to the room to weigh and measure her, put in eye drops, and give a vitamin K shot. After all these procedures were completed, the nurse commented, very matter-of-factly, that she was going to do a heel prick and test her blood sugar levels. I asked why she would do that, and she stated that it was because my daughter was shaking a bit. (I'm pretty sure that after being somewhere really warm and snug for nine months and then having a stranger poke and prod me as I lay naked and helpless, I would likely be shivering as well.) I told her I did not want it done and she pushed the issue a bit. In a breastfeeding friendly hospital, breastfeeding would be, in most cases, the suggested next step if a baby had low blood sugar, so why not allow the baby to continue to be with her mother and continue to nurse if breast-feeding had already been successfully initiated? There were no other red flags or high risk histories to suggest anything more serious, so why create a situation that in many cases would lead to the suggestion to offer a bottle of formula to increase the baby's blood sugar, undermine a mother's confidence, interfere with the natural process of breastfeeding, and alter a baby's gut flora and ability to fend off foreign pathogens? After a few moments of my demanding she not do the test and that she give my daughter back to me, the nurse did return my daughter, but I'll always remember the feeling of helplessness I felt in that situation and the understanding I gained about how a new mother can feel when confronted with the strong opinions of medical staff.

These types of unnecessary interventions are common: inductions that are done to speed up the process instead of trusting in nature's schedule, c-sections because of the fear that the baby is too big, narcotics used for pain management that slow down labour or impact the body's natural endorphin release, separation of mom and baby immediately following delivery traumatizing a baby and interfering with the normal bonding process that follows birth. Do you see the pattern here? Interventions that have the potential to affect breastfeeding are ones that somehow impact the natural, biological process and continuum. Beginning to look at the process as a continuum will help you determine what may cause negative effects and which interventions are less perilous to the breastfeeding relationship.

Below you will find a number of common birth interventions and brief explanations of how they may affect breastfeeding.

Induction/Pitocin—Induction of labour with the use of pitocin has the potential to prolong labour. Pitocin is a synthetic form of oxytocin which you will recall is the hormone that stimulates contractions during labour. Pitocin, however, does not have the same impact on our bodies as does natural oxytocin. Unlike oxytocin, pitocin does not cross the blood-brain barrier which means it has no impact on our brains or on our emotions. You'll also remember that oxytocin is known as the "love hormone" due to its impact on bonding and, when present in conjunction with prolactin, causes mothering instincts. Synthetic pitocin gives none of these benefits.[10]

Anytime an induction is begun, a mother begins a process of monitoring and often is confined to bed. The more monitoring that is done, the greater the possibility that other interventions will be started as medical staff interpret what their monitors are telling them. And being confined to bed has the potential to slow the process of labour as the mother no longer benefits from movement to both speed labour and help with pain management. In terms of pain management, pitocin often brings on very strong contractions that are consistent in strength, unlike natural contractions that slowly build. For this reason, inductions often are closely followed by epidurals. And following this potential to slow labour and increase pain, there is a higher risk of labour ending in a c-section.

Induction can lead to a delay in milk production due to the lengthy IV use which can cause a decrease in serum prolactin levels. IV fluids can increase edema and engorgement which can have a detrimental effect on the mother's comfort and newborn's ability to latch on. Pitocin is also an anti-diuretic which causes the body to retain more fluids and can lead to increased engorgement.

IV Fluids—Lengthy use of IV fluids can introduce a large amount of fluid into a mother's system. These fluids can dilute the prolactin in the blood stream which in turn can affect the lactation process, sometimes delaying milk production. Excess fluids can also cause increased swelling and engorgement making latching on difficult for a baby. If there is glucose in the IV fluids, the glucose keeps mom's and baby's blood sugar levels abnormally high. The body makes extra insulin to combat the high sugar levels and, once the baby is born and glucose is cut off, extra insulin can result in hypoglycemia (low blood sugar). Following delivery, this can then lead to numerous interventions that have the potential to separate mom and baby and can cause unnecessary stress on the baby.

C-Section—A c-section has the potential to separate mom and baby which limits the opportunity to breastfeed within the first hour or so after delivery. This window is very important and can never be recaptured. The pain from the incision site can cause a mother difficulty in caring for and holding her baby. The baby may also be affected by pain medications given to the mother during the surgery. Charlotte, who ended up with a c-section after thirty-six hours of labour, says that she "was completely numb both physically and emotionally" and that she did not "feel any of the new mom feelings of sadness, elation, or relief." Her experience indicates that c-sections can affect not only the physical aspect of breastfeeding, but they have the potential to affect the emotional aspects as well. If you have an unscheduled c-section, you may find that you need to work through the emotions surrounding your experience. Often moms will feel that they have "missed out" on the normal delivery experience and just as when breastfeeding doesn't work out, women who have a c-section may need to grieve the loss of what was expected.

Epidurals — Epidurals stop a mother's release of endorphins which are the body's natural painkillers. These endorphins are also passed along to a newborn through the mother's milk following delivery. If a mother has had an epidural, the baby does not have the benefit of these natural painkillers to help with any pain or discomfort the baby may feel after the birth process. Epidurals also increase the likelihood of a longer labour — and thereby increase the likelihood of a c-section, increase the risk of malpositioning due to bed confinement, and increase the risk of pitocin use. Epidurals also increase the risk of neonatal jaundice since a baby's liver, which must break down bilirubin, must now also break down the drugs from the epidural that have passed through from the mother to baby. (Bilirubin is created by the normal breakdown of red blood cells. It is excreted as bile in stool. High levels of bilirubin in the blood may cause jaundice.) Epidurals, or any other drugs used during labour, increase this load on a baby's liver.

There is some controversy over the direct effect of epidurals on breastfeeding but studies have shown decreased neonatal suckling ability, increased risk of bottle supplementation, and decreased serum oxytocin levels in the mother and have shown that babies born to moms who received epidurals have more difficulty breastfeeding in the early days after birth and are weaned earlier — they are more than twice as likely to wean within the first six months compared to women with no epidural.[11,12] One such study done by Baumgarder, Muehl, Fischer, and Pribbenow concluded that "Labor epidural anesthesia had a negative impact on breast-feeding in the first 24 hours of life even though it did not inhibit the percentage of breast-feeding attempts in the first hour."[13] The drugs used in epidurals can make a baby drowsy and inhibit a baby's reflex responses. An epidural also means an IV for the mother, and often a urinary catheter, electronic fetal monitoring, and blood pressure monitoring.

Pain Management/Analgesia—Some of the drugs used for pain management include Nubain, Stadol, and nitrous oxide gas (laughing gas). These drugs do cross the placenta. Drugs taken for pain can therefore affect a baby's ability to breastfeed. These drugs have the potential to decrease alertness, decrease respiration, decrease sucking, decrease responsiveness, and lower Apgar scores, which can affect the baby's after-care. If pain management must be used, it is best if used as close to delivery as possible to lessen the amount of drugs that cross the placenta and enter the baby's system, or a few hours prior to delivery to allow the mother's liver time to metabolize the drugs. Due to babies' immature renal and liver functions, it takes babies longer to clear drugs from their systems than it would an adult.

Prolonged Labour—A prolonged labour can influence a doctor's management of labour and delivery and increase the risk of caesarean birth and other interventions.

Birth Trauma—Birth trauma can include such interventions as the use of forceps, vacuum, or suctioning. These types of interventions can cause trauma, oral aversion, and pain which may affect a baby's ability to breastfeed.

After-Care of Baby and Mom—Immediate after-care of a baby following delivery (washing, weighing, injections, heel pricks, eye ointments, etc.) separate mom and baby and can stress a baby and cause a baby to enter a parasympathetic state. This means that a baby "shuts down." There are few options for a newborn when faced with an outward stressor. They can't fight and they can't run, but they can withdraw and shut down.

Early bathing before a baby has the opportunity to breastfeed can have a negative impact on breastfeeding. A baby uses scent and taste to find the nipple. Videos of newborns crawling to the breast, locating the nipple, and latching on show that babies repeatedly pause, suck on their fists and then continue. It is hypothesized that perhaps the scent and taste on their hands from the amniotic fluid is similar to their mother's nipple and this scent assists them in locating the breast and latching on successfully. It is apparent that babies who are first bathed before being allowed to seek out the breast show a decreased success in locating the breast on their own and latching on successfully.

In most situations, there is no harm in waiting until after the first feed for *all* baby care: bathing, weighing, vitamin K shot, eye ointment, pictures, etc. In some circumstances where a baby's health is in immediate danger or the conditions of delivery present a potential risk to the baby, it will be necessary to assess the baby's condition immediately. However, you can request the baby not be cleaned or treatments such as eye ointment be delayed until you have had a chance to be with your baby for awhile.

With respect to mom's after-care, it is important to remember that babies are working on innate knowledge and instinct. As mentioned above, one of the feedback mechanisms a baby uses to organize feeding and recognize mom as mom is the mother's scent. Having a shower too soon after delivery, before the baby has had a chance to establish breastfeeding, may introduce new scents and wash off a mother's natural scent affecting her baby's ability to find the breast and latch. As wonderful as that first shower is after delivery, it's best to first wait for breastfeeding to get established.

Circumcision—Circumcision is not done as routinely as it once was. The choice to circumcise your son is a personal and cultural choice. It is important to realize though that it can in some cases have an effect on breastfeeding. Pain causes disorganization and can therefore affect a baby's ability to suck. It can cause withdrawal and send the baby into a deep sleep which may interfere with your baby's need to feed frequently. If you decide to have your son circumcised, consider waiting until after feeding is established and demand that the doctor use some type of pain control during and after the procedure. Allowing your baby to breastfeed as soon as the procedure is complete, and ensuring your baby can breastfeed as often as desired after the procedure, will help to lessen the effect of the procedure.

Supplementation—Supplementation with formula has a consistently negative bearing on breastfeeding durations. Supplementation use can result in reduced breastfeeding durations.[14] The reasons for this may be a direct result of the supplementation, the reduction in the frequency of breastfeeding and resulting drop in milk supply, but they may also be a result of a mother's views and parenting philosophy.

It should be noted that there are very specific guidelines that some hospitals follow in determining when supplementation is appropriate. In Canada, for example, the Breastfeeding Committee for Canada has developed the *Guidelines for WHO/UNICEF Baby-Friendly™ Initiative (BFI) in Canada*. The guidelines look at two specific groups of babies. The first group is babies who are ill, in need of surgery, or are of very low birth weight. It is recognized that these babies will have special needs and each babies' feeding needs will be determined on an individual basis.

For newborns who are with their mothers, the document indicates there are "very few indications for supplements." The situations in which a baby may require supplementation are listed as:

- infants whose mothers are severely ill,
- infants with inborn errors of metabolism,
- infants with acute water loss, and
- infants whose mothers are taking medication which is contraindicated when breastfeeding.[15]

And in all cases, breast milk is the recommended type of supplementation whenever possible and mothers are encouraged to use a breast pump to initiate and maintain their milk supply until direct breastfeeding may begin or continue.

Interruption of the Birthing Process—The birth process requires privacy. In order for the process to progress normally, a mother needs to feel safe and secure. When a mother's privacy is compromised, labour often slows or stops completely. The reasons for this can be found in our evolutionary path and the needs of our ancestors. Consider a peaceful forest scene. A doe is in the beginning stages of labour. She finds a quiet place to rest as her labour progresses. Suddenly, the doe senses the presence of a wolf and she begins to stir. Her labour slows, and then stops as she moves to a different location far away from the threat of a predator. Once she feels safe again, her labour continues and her fawn is born shortly thereafter. This situation is no different than what's experienced by many women in a hospital birthing environment.

When a mother feels afraid, insecure, or overly-anxious, adrenaline is released in her body. Endorphins occur naturally during labour and are intended to ease the pain and give a somewhat euphoric feeling. But when adrenaline is present, it works against this process. Kroeger explains that "With poor pain control and increased fear and anxiety, adrenaline works as an antagonist to oxytocin, weakens uterine contractions, prolongs labor, and may set the stage for IV oxytocin augmentation, medical pain relief, possible restriction to bed, electronic monitoring, and the possibility that an instrumental delivery or cesarean section will be performed."[16] For this reason, it is important for a mother to feel secure, calm, and have a sense of being alone and private during labour.

If you consider the environment in most hospitals' labour and delivery rooms it is anything but private and secure. There is plenty of noise from outside the room; nurses, doctors, medical students, and other staff come and go without much concern for your comfort level or privacy; you are inundated with questions, often at inopportune times; and you are expected to bare yourself for seemingly every person who enters the room without concern for your comfort and often without much of an introduction. In short, most birth experiences in hospitals provide very little in the way of privacy and security. So what is the impact? It can be as dramatic as the doe who is confronted by a predator. Often labour slows or stops altogether. If a mother is not comfortable in her environment, or doesn't feel safe, it can have a very strong impact on the progression of labour.

Consider your own labour or the experiences of friends. A common story is of a woman who begins labour at home, then goes to the hospital and suddenly labour seemingly stops. At this point, women are often sent home or doctors decide that pitocin is necessary to move the process along. Failure to progress is a common reason given to women when pitocin or even c-sections are recommended. Of course, these interventions are sometimes necessary, but in some cases, the true cause of the failure to progress has little to do with the mother's inability to move through the process of childbirth and more to do with the lack of privacy and security afforded in a medicalized setting.

When entering the hospital setting, ensure you have someone with you who can advocate on your behalf. Have your advocate speak for you and work to maintain a quiet, peaceful room; limit the people who enter your room; question tests or procedures that may be recommended; and help to protect your privacy and modesty. During labour is not the time you need to be fighting for your rights or feeling uncomfortable, so have someone with you who can do all that for you allowing you to focus on what's important: birthing your baby.

Birth Process and Bonding and Breastfeeding— The Continuum

Numerous times throughout the first section of this book I have mentioned the idea of a continuum between birth and breastfeeding. It is important to recognize that as mothers we begin nurturing and nourishing our babies from the moment of conception. The way in which we nurture and nourish our children may change from pregnancy to post-pregnancy to weaning, but there is no moment when we stop nourishing or nurturing our children. To recognize this continuum is important in understanding the biological nature of how we mother, and this recognition will help us to make choices that work with the continuum instead of fighting against it.

From the moment of our baby's conception, our bodies go through remarkable changes to allow for the pregnancy to proceed and to prepare our bodies for the awesome job of creating and nourishing a baby within our womb. And it truly is an awesome feat! But our amazing abilities do not end with childbirth. Our bodies are also created to nourish and nurture our babies at our breasts following delivery. Breastfeeding not only provides for the nutritional requirements of an infant, it also meets many of the emotional and physical needs of a baby. As our bodies prepare to birth our babies, beginning their life in the world, our bodies are also preparing for an initial bonding experience between ourselves and our babies, as well as ensuring breastfeeding, the means of providing nourishment, is established in as effective a manner as possible.

As our bodies prepare for childbirth, our hormone levels are changing preparing us for lactation and motherhood. As discussed earlier in this chapter, the most important hormones at play are prolactin and oxytocin. Prolactin is the hormone that allows lactation and also creates mothering instincts, and oxytocin is the hormone that causes contractions during labour, initiates the milk ejection response when breastfeeding, and is known as the hormone of love. When these two hormones are present together, they encourage bonding between mom and baby.

Immediately following delivery, both oxytocin and prolactin are present at extremely high levels. This helps to bridge the continuum between pregnancy and the post-partum period. Oxytocin is flooding the brain in a wash of good feelings, and the object of our affection at this point is, hopefully, our newborn. When our new baby latches and nurses immediately after delivery, a wave of oxytocin is released and passed to our baby. This begins the bonding between mom and baby. This is one reason why certain interventions that affect the levels of prolactin or oxytocin in a mother's system can affect the initial bonding between mom and baby and also the initiation of breastfeeding. Ideally, to avoid any potentially negative impact, it is best to avoid those interventions that may affect the natural hormones in a mother's system. But this isn't always possible. What is possible in almost all cases is skin-to-skin quiet time between mom and baby following delivery. Be sure to make your wishes known to the hospital staff with regards to your desire for immediate skin-to-skin time with your baby following delivery.

The Importance of the First Feed

In order to benefit from the high levels of oxytocin and prolactin following delivery, and make use of the innate skills and reflexes with which babies are born, it is very important to initiate breastfeeding soon after delivery. This time is one of relief (your baby has safely arrived), excitement (your baby has safely arrived), and discovery (your baby has safely arrived). It is recommended that a baby be allowed to nurse within the first hour following birth, and in a normal delivery, babies will usually seek out the breast and can even latch on their own within the first hour and often much sooner.

This is a period of importance for the mother as well as the baby. Mary Kroeger and Linda Smith in their book, *Impact of Birthing Practices on Breastfeeding*, explain that just as there is a sensitive period for the newborn following birth, so too is there "a similar 'sensitive period' for the mother, during which she too is 'looking' for her newborn and is receptive to the first feed."[17] This first hour of life is critical for both mother and baby and should be cherished and protected. Kroeger and Smith later explain, "This first 60 minutes are critical, and a vast body of science on imprinting in other mammals suggests that timing can determine the whole future of mothering."[18] So while the importance of the first hour or so of life, and the timing of the first feed, are important to the bonding of mother and baby as well as the establishment of breastfeeding, understanding the importance is also critical to assist you in making decisions and creating an environment that will help rather than hinder your breastfeeding efforts.

This doesn't mean that you need to force your baby to nurse. No, indeed, enjoy the first moments after your baby's birth as a time to relax, explore your new baby, share the joy with your partner, and snuggle the baby that you have thought about and dreamed of over the past nine months. Keep your baby with you, skin-to-skin, covered with a warm blanket. Your body will keep your baby warm. Delay all procedures that are not time-sensitive until you and your baby have had some quiet time and your baby has had the opportunity to nurse. For full-term, healthy babies these procedures include weighing, cleaning, blood tests, injections, and eye drops. Babies who have had normal deliveries will begin to move towards the breast, crawling and searching. You can certainly assist your baby into a position to nurse, but do trust their ability. You will be amazed at your baby's ability to do much of it on their own. Ultimately, we as mothers need to learn to work with our babies, assist them in what they need to do, and learn not to interfere with their natural instincts and reflexes.

This early interaction between mother and baby is an important part of the continuum. Not only will the baby get an initial dose of colostrum which will provide many benefits, but this early experience begins the bonding process making use of the high hormone levels present following delivery. Not to mention that after nine months of carrying your baby and potentially hours of labour, the opportunity to share some quiet moments cuddling with your baby and beginning your baby's life in a relaxing, loving, safe way is one that you really don't want to miss.

But what if your baby is born via c-section or interventions such as pain control or the use of pitocin are unavoidable in your case? These things may make the initial breastfeeding experience a little more challenging, but the closeness of skin-to-skin contact and uninterrupted time with your baby following a difficult delivery are all the more important. Variation from what would be considered "normal" birth does not mean all hope has been lost. Instead, see these unexpected interventions as motivation for following through with an initial first feed and skin-to-skin contact in order to counteract, as much as possible, the negative impact from the interventions. It is not always possible to avoid birth interventions or follow what would be considered a normal birthing pattern, but we should always seek to rebalance our experience according to the biologically normal pattern of birth and breastfeeding. Deviations will always occur, unexpectedly and unavoidably, but always try to recentre yourself and your baby and return to what would be considered biologically normal. Even small changes can have a big impact. Don't think you have to do everything "just so". Everything helps and those small changes might be the key to breastfeeding success for you and your baby. It's not always possible to have everything follow the biologically normal process; do what you can.

The Importance of Skin-to-Skin Contact

Skin-to-skin contact, or close proximity, is important not only immediately following delivery but continuing through your baby's first months. Skin-to-skin contact helps keep babies calm. Don't forget that you were your baby's home for nine months. Being as close to you as possible is comforting to a baby and brings a sense of security and relaxation. Close contact with mom also assists a baby in regulating his or her own body temperature, respiration, and heart rate. For mom, there is nothing like taking time to relax and snuggle with your baby. It's good for your state of mind, forces you to slow down and focus on what is really important, raises prolactin levels which help milk production, and can give you the peace of mind that you are capable of calming your baby and meeting your baby's needs.

Skin-to-skin contact is not only of benefit in the early hours and days post-partum; it can also benefit mom and baby at any stage. If you are having breastfeeding difficulties, placing your baby skin-to-skin in a reclined position with your baby snuggled on your chest can assist your baby to utilize the reflexes and skills with which he or she was born and return to a more primal pattern based on innate skills rather than learned behaviours. It can also help both mom and baby to simply relax and trust in the process.

Skin-to-skin contact is also a very valuable strategy to use if your baby is born prematurely. When used with premature babies, skin-to-skin care is known as kangaroo mother care or KMC and is a wonderful way to participate in your baby's care, spend time bonding with your new baby, and benefit your baby's health and growth.[19]

Mothering from a Biological Perspective

> When a baby cries inconsolably for hours, when its tiny body arches in frustration, when its fists punch the air in anger, we see the clearest example of the clash between biology and culture.
>
> —Meredith Small, Professor of Anthropology, Cornell University[20]

This quote by Meredith Small sums up the challenges of mothers today. We are caught in an impossible position between our culture and our biology and we struggle to balance the two. Our biology cries out to us to keep our babies close, respond to them when they cry, and allow them to sleep near us at night so we are aware of their needs and can attend to them quickly. Our culture suggests that babies should have their own place to rest away from us (think bouncy chairs, baby swings, play pens, car seats), that picking them up every time they cry will only spoil them and make them needy, and that a baby must be trained early on to sleep in his or her own bed and usually in a separate room. Our babies are born expecting closeness and responsiveness, but our culture tells us this isn't what is right or accepted. What is a mother to do?[21]

More and more I think mothers are beginning to respond from a biological place. More parents are babywearing and keeping their babies close. More parents are choosing to co-sleep or have their baby in close proximity to them at night in a crib. And more parents are choosing to quickly respond to their babies' cries believing that young infants are not manipulative or demanding but are instead legitimately in need of closeness and connection with their parents.

This isn't to say that parents who choose to keep their babies sitting in bouncy chairs or in their own bedrooms, or who choose not to respond whenever their babies cry are choosing not to meet the needs of their infants or attempting to train their babies to be independent at an early age. But it is often our culture and society making these choices instead of biology. What does biology suggest when it comes to the care of young infants?

It suggests, as described above, that babies be kept close. While mom is always important to a baby, it doesn't have to be only mom who maintains this closeness. Other caregivers such as the father, grandparents, or even older siblings can carry a baby or maintain proximity. This proximity allows for quick response when a baby indicates a need. And for older infants, the inclusion of the baby in daily activities such as shopping, housework, or gardening—and from the perspective of the mother or caregiver as opposed to the lower perspective offered by a stroller or car seat—allows the baby to experience the world and learn about social interactions and the boundaries and expectations of daily life.

Biology also suggests that babies be responded to when they indicate that they have a need. There is some suggestion that a baby's cry is particularly sharp and piercing in order to elicit the necessary response from its parents. Babies who are able to make themselves heard receive attention quicker than babies who are not heard. A cry is a call for help. It is not intended as manipulation or entertainment. Responding to your baby's cry meets his or her needs, teaches your baby that he or she is safe and secure, and, let's face it, helps you maintain your sanity.

These two aspects of biology are particularly important when it comes to initiating breastfeeding. Our society's attitudes towards, and instruction about, breastfeeding are all too often based on a view of formula feeding being the norm. If we breastfeed from this norm, we risk harming the breastfeeding relationship. If we are to follow biological principles for breastfeeding, it is important to learn to trust our own mothering instincts, trust our babies' instincts and indications of need, keep our babies close, and respond to our babies early and always.

Trusting your own mothering instincts can be one of the most challenging aspects of mothering. We are conditioned to follow the rules, and our society has created lots of rules for mothers. Don't pick up your baby too much or it'll be spoiled. Never let your baby use the breast for comfort. Don't sleep with your baby or you'll never get your baby into his or her own bed. Do you think mother dogs or horses have these rules? I doubt it! They trust their own instincts and do what comes naturally. It can be difficult, I admit, to push away all the information with which we are bombarded or the good-natured and well-meaning advice given to us by family, but motherhood is as good a time as any to stand up for what it is you want to do and to follow your own lead when it comes to your baby.

Learning to trust your baby's instincts can be equally difficult. Generations have looked at infants as manipulative and needing to be controlled and trained. It makes little sense from a biological perspective for a baby to be this way. Indeed, babies are born with a wide range of reflexes and instincts which are there to ensure their survival. Sucking, crying, seeking the breast and latching, grasping: all of these reflexes and many more are part of your baby's amazing repertoire at birth. Babies also have the knowledge of when they need to eat, how much they need to eat, when they need to sleep, and what makes them feel secure. Trust your baby. And in conjunction with trusting your baby, learn to trust your baby through the lens of your own mothering instincts. In combination, you have an amazing store of knowledge that will take you a very long way.

In order to learn to trust your baby's innate skills and your own instincts, it is important that you keep your baby close. Those early feeding cues are subtle and can be missed if you are always across the room or having someone else care for the baby who isn't in tune with a baby's cues. Don't get me wrong; I know as mothers we need some time to ourselves. In the early days and weeks, a shower all to ourselves can feel like a week at the spa! But learning how to live your life and integrate your baby into it will be a great benefit not only to your breastfeeding relationship, but to your own sanity. Babywearing is a wonderful way to make it possible to keep your baby nearby in order to respond quickly to her needs. Wraps, mei tais, slings, pouches, or structured carriers can all be used as comfortable and convenient carriers. When you're not carrying your baby, ensure that you can still be in a position to respond to her needs. If you have other caregivers helping with the care of your infant, ensure they understand the early feeding cues and are prepared to bring the baby to you if she indicates a need to nurse.[22]

Keeping your baby close is not just about meeting your baby's needs; it is very important to initiating and maintaining your milk supply. As discussed earlier, frequent nursing is critical in the early days to establish lactation and set production. Having your baby close by makes frequent nursing much more likely. It is easy for a baby to indicate a need to nurse and then simply fall back to sleep if that cue is not caught. A baby who is not nursing well may simply not have the energy to signal its need in a more obvious way, but if you have your baby close to you, you can respond to those early cues. Aside from the benefits to lactation, by having your baby close and responding quickly to early feeding cues and indications of other needs, you will have a baby who cries much less and this is of course of benefit to everyone in the house!

Keeping your baby close is directly connected to responding to your baby's needs early and often. So often in our society there is information about scheduling infant feeding or training your baby to sleep at an early age. This type of information is all too often based on formula feeding and is counter to breastfeeding practices. Because a mother's milk supply is individual to her and her baby, there is no one-size-fits-all schedule that can be followed. Storage capacity also is individual and has a large impact on how often a baby needs to nurse. If we try to manage our babies' schedules, we end up interfering with the natural process of lactation and risk affecting our supply, often negatively. Responding to your baby's cues is critical to establishing and maintaining milk supply. Trusting your baby's own ability to know when he needs to eat, and how much he needs to eat, actually frees us as mothers. We don't need to have control over our babies' schedules. Instead we only have to provide what is needed when it is needed.

It's all well and good to say that you need to respond to your baby, meet his needs, keep him close and trust both yourself and your baby, but when confronted with the messages from our culture and society it can be difficult to follow through with this. We'll talk more in an upcoming chapter about building your support structure and dealing with conflicting advice from friends and family, but for now, let's just say that one of the most important things you can do to ensure your success is, as has been said all along, to educate yourself. We cannot remove ourselves from our society or culture, but we most certainly can choose not to follow it unquestioningly. If we choose to look at pregnancy, birth, and breastfeeding from a biological perspective, we will begin to view these events through a new lens. You will begin to see alternative choices and possibilities. If you are educated, you can begin to make decisions that will work best for you, but also decisions that will not work against the biological aspects of breastfeeding.

Importance of Mother's Health

Since it is not commonly discussed, I think it is important here to mention that there are a number of health issues that can affect breastfeeding. You can't always remove conditions that will potentially affect breastfeeding, but if you are not aware of the potential for complications, it is impossible to try to mediate their effects or make efforts to remove the risk prior to getting pregnant or prior to delivery.

Mother's Weight

Being overweight is often linked to difficulties in conceiving and pregnancy, but excess weight in a mother is also related to difficulties with lactation. Obesity increases the likelihood of birth interventions such as prolonged labour and c-sections. But obesity also has a direct impact on breastfeeding. Statistically, overweight mothers are less likely to initiate breastfeeding and are more likely to wean early. Lactogenesis II can be delayed in mothers who are overweight and the prolactin response is weakened.[23,24]

Cigarette Smoking

There are numerous reasons why, if you are a smoker before pregnancy, you should quit smoking, but one that may not be commonly recognized is that smoking can decrease a mother's milk supply and delay lactogenesis II.[25] Early weaning has been associated with a mother's smoking. Mothers who smoke before, during, and after pregnancy are 2.18 times more likely not to breastfeed at all and those who continue to smoke after the birth of their baby are 2.3-2.4 times more likely to have weaned before ten weeks.[26] If you are a smoker, quitting is obviously the best option for everyone involved. Nicotine patches have been shown to be quite safe for a breastfeeding infant and may be an option for you.[27] Infants whose mothers were using a nicotine patch received significantly less nicotine than did those with smoking mothers and would also be protected from the environmental harm caused by cigarette smoking, including increased risk of asthma and respiratory problems and even behavioural and academic concerns.[28,29,30]

Diabetes

Mothers with type I diabetes are most definitely encouraged to breastfeed. Indeed, breastfeeding may lessen the symptoms of diabetes and potentially reduce the risk of the baby developing diabetes. However, it is important to realize that diabetes can delay lactogenesis II. This is a result of lower prolactin concentrations in mothers with diabetes compared to mothers who do not have diabetes. Mothers with diabetes are encouraged to begin pumping or hand expressing as soon as possible to encourage milk production.[31]

Polycystic Ovarian Syndrome (PCOS)

Due to the hormonal imbalances caused by PCOS, breastfeeding can often be challenging. While many women with PCOS have no difficulty breastfeeding, milk production is often affected. While breastfeeding can be possible, some women with PCOS have difficulty establishing a full milk supply. Some medications such as metformin and domperidone can be used and herbal remedies such as alfalfa leaf, red raspberry leaf, or nettle can sometimes help.[32] It is most important that women with PCOS understand how this syndrome can affect lactation and that they prepare for these potential challenges early on in pregnancy by gathering information, discussing options with a doctor and lactation consultant, and putting in place a strong support system. Surprisingly, one-third of women with PCOS will experience extreme over-supply which brings with it its own set of challenges.[33] Again, planning for lactation during pregnancy with the help of a knowledgeable, supportive doctor and lactation consultant can help prepare you for potential issues related to PCOS.[34]

Thyroid Disease

Thyroid issues can arise during and after pregnancy. Hypothyroidism can affect a mother's milk supply since the thyroid has a role in the initiation of milk supply. If your thyroid levels are already low, or borderline, this may affect your supply. Common symptoms of hypothyroidism include an enlarged thyroid, sensitivity to cold, dry skin, excessive hair loss, and fatigue. If you are concerned, see your doctor to have your thyroid checked. Treatment is simple and compatible with breastfeeding.

Hypoplastic Breasts

In a perfect world, doctors and obstetricians would do breast exams for women during their pregnancies and would indicate if there is anything that might affect a woman's breastfeeding efforts. Rarely are women told they have hypoplastic breasts or that this condition can have a bearing on the ability to produce sufficient quantities of milk for their babies.

"Hypoplastic breasts" refers to a lack of breast tissue. This is different from simply having small breasts. Women with hypoplastic breasts often do not develop glandular breast tissue to any great extent during puberty and often do not undergo normal breast changes during pregnancy. While a lack of breast tissue prior to pregnancy does not mean a woman *will* have problems with milk production, it does warrant careful monitoring and additional consideration after the birth of the baby. It is also advisable to see a lactation consultant prior to the birth of your baby (even prior to getting pregnant if possible) to see about possible treatments or protocols that could be used. The use of progesterone, for example, may promote breast development during pregnancy. PCOS and insufficient glandular tissue are often linked.[35]

Knowing you have hypoplastic breasts prior to the birth of your baby is an important first step in mitigating its effects and working towards breastfeeding, even if only partial breastfeeding. Ask your doctor to do a breast exam or see a lactation consultant early in your pregnancy to rule out or diagnose hypoplastic breasts if you have any concerns.

Breast Surgery or Trauma

Previous breast surgery or other traumas to the breast can cause difficulties with breastfeeding. Breast reduction surgery carries the greatest risk, but other surgeries such as augmentation and lifts and other diagnostic procedures can possibly impact a mother's milk supply. For more information see Diane West's book *Defining Your Own Success* (2001) .

Charlotte's Story

With my first pregnancy I was more or less ambivalent about breastfeeding, assuming that I would try it and like it. It wasn't on my radar of potential problems that could happen with a newborn. I was more worried about SIDS than any potential breastfeeding problems. After delivery the new and most challenging part of infant parenting started for me and my husband, namely, how was I going to feed this baby?

After a gruelling thirty-six hour labour and c-section, I gave birth to my first child, a baby girl named Annika. I was completely numb both physically and emotionally. I did not feel any of the new mom feelings of sadness, elation, or relief. I remained completely numb for the first few days of my daughter's life. She was brought to me at regular intervals for feeding, but it soon became apparent that she was not sucking at all. She would scream and pull away every single time I tried to nurse her. I had many lactation consultants come around during all hours of the night and day trying to get her to latch. We tried the Lact-Aid nursing system, nipple shields, and many other devices in order to try to get the latch. We left the hospital with formula, but were still trying hard to breastfeed with the help of an off-site lactation consultant. We had several appointments that ended with no latch.

Finally, two weeks after her birth, a dear friend of mine came over and brought me her Pump in Style. She was desperately worried about my daughter because of her inability to suck and my daughter wasn't getting much of anything from the Lact-Aid system. I pumped six ounces, which was such a relief to me, knowing that I was actually making milk. I will never forget the look on my daughter's face when I gave her that first bottle of pumped breast milk. The nipple went in with her screaming red in the face, but after a few seconds she completely relaxed, her body went limp and her eyes rolled to the back of her head. She drank the entire six ounces and fell into a deep sleep. I had finally fed her, and so began a year of pumping that I still regard with gratitude and a bit of disdain. It was hard. It nearly drove me nuts. But it was good for my girl.

For about six months after her birth I continued daily to put her to the breast in an attempt to get her interested in it again. But each time she reacted the same as she had in the first moments after she was born—she screamed until she was red in the face and pulled away. So after about six months, I gave up trying and resigned myself to the idea that it was just never going to happen.

I do think that my daughter's inability to breastfeed contributed to my post-partum depression, which lasted only a month. It was the most difficult part of our newborn experience, and now, because I have been able to breastfeed my second baby, I fully realize the loss of that breastfeeding relationship. Back then, I couldn't have known what I was missing, but now when I lie down to nurse my son, I see clearly what I missed with my daughter. Even though there is a loss, it also makes me realize how resilient our children are. Our rough start is part of our story and I'm not even sure I would change it if I could.

Before I gave birth to my second child, I assumed I would have problems, and I did. I actually was unable to get a latch again, and after a week of poor latching went right to the pump. At five months of age my son was ready and able to breastfeed and one long weekend we made the transition from the pump to the breast and it was heavenly! It took my body about a week to wean off of the pump completely because I was overproducing with the pump, but we soon fell into a rhythm and I haven't touched the pump since.

The most frustrating part of my experience with pumping was not getting any answers as to why both of my babies had trouble nursing. At the time my daughter was born I had a lot of friends who were really into attachment parenting and they made me feel just awful about not being able to nurse her. They would make comments suggesting that I had given up too easily and that if I had just stuck with it another week, she would have latched. Even though I knew this was not true, I was vulnerable, as all first-time moms are, and I ended up thinking that maybe they were right. Could it be that I had given up too easily? I am now confident that I played *no* part in my children's inability to nurse and that were it not for my pumping efforts they would not have gotten any breast milk at all.

I was also unable to get any answers from the lactation consultants, my pediatrician, or the hospital staff. Nobody knew why my daughter couldn't latch. After I started pumping and giving breast milk through the bottle, I noticed that she was having difficulty with the bottle. She would pull away and cry all the time and the milk would pour down the sides of her mouth and she wasn't getting much. I was referred to a newborn occupational therapist who diagnosed her with an oral delay. This terrified us and we wondered if it would affect her speech (it didn't). After many expensive, fancy bottles, which included the Haberman feeder, she got better, at around six months of age.

With my son, I knew what to do and was more confident in pumping, so it was easier and less bewildering. I still saw at least three different lactation consultants, none of whom had any experience with this sort of breastfeeding trouble and they could not tell me why he was not able to latch.

My second child is now almost a year old and is nursing like a pro. I am so grateful for the opportunity to nurse him and I know it will carry us to places we might not otherwise have gone. Being able to nurse my second baby has healed many of the hurts left over from having to pump for my first. If you are pregnant for the second time, it is worth trying to nurse a second baby.

Create Your Experience

"Being able to nurse my second baby has healed many of the hurts
left over from having to pump for my first."

Charlotte, mom of two

S uccess and failure. What do they really mean? As discussed in a previous chapter, part of success means
defining what success is to you. As you begin to consider
the possibilities of breastfeeding a new baby, allow yourself to
consider what success will mean for you. Do not plan your
expectations, but instead plan your success. Recognize that rarely
in life do things go as we expect them to go. But we always have
choices; we always have the ability to react to the experiences we
are given. You may not have had the experience you had hoped
for breastfeeding your first baby, but you can determine if you
will be successful the next time around. The first step is recognizing that you have choices and control. You may not always be
able to control what happens, but you can control how you react.
If you are faced with a c-section, for example, you can choose
how you will interact with your baby, how you will manage
lactation to give you and your baby the best possible chance of
success, and how you will determine your own success.

In this chapter, we'll pull together many of the elements from
the book which can be important to achieving a positive breastfeeding experience. There is no sure-fire plan to make breastfeed-

ing a success, but through education, support, and perseverance you can greatly increase the likelihood that you and your baby will establish a close breastfeeding relationship. We'll first briefly discuss emotions, then move on to the importance of learning to trust in your body again, the value of information and support systems, how expectations play into our experience, and finally, the biological process of breastfeeding, mothering, and bonding.

An Emotional Journey

Emotions are an integral part of our human experience but it is important to understand how to handle emotions and not be controlled by them. Acknowledge and then *move on*. Motherhood is an emotional time. We are so closely tied to our babies, both emotionally and physically, and want only to do what is best for them. When confronted with the constant chatter of society, friends, family, and the chatter in our own heads, it is easy to become overwhelmed and overly emotional. Breastfeeding only serves to make these emotions all the more raw, and it is common for new mothers to see breastfeeding problems as the source of all the emotional upheaval. Rarely is this the case.

I fell into this trap myself when my daughter was born. I was already emotional and on edge given my challenges breastfeeding my son and feared that the second time around things still wouldn't work out as I hoped. Going into the experience, I was determined to do everything I could to make choices that would help to encourage breastfeeding and bonding. My daughter nursed for the first time within about a half hour of her birth, nursed frequently during her stay in the hospital, was well over her birth weight at only six days of age, and continued to be an eager nurser. But after about two weeks she was crying a lot, nursing frequently, and I had suffered through engorgement. I was well aware of the process of lactation, breastfeeding management, and newborn behaviour, but even though she was gaining weight exceedingly well and was a happy baby—as long as she was moving or being held—I went through a period of self-doubt thinking *I* wasn't going to be able to make breastfeeding work for us; *I* would be a failure yet again.

In reality, my daughter was just experiencing a difficult adjustment to her fourth trimester.[1] It is very likely that she would have gone through the same difficult period if she had been bottle-fed, and it is likely that it would have been even worse without the comfort of nursing and the close physical contact she craved. But it is instructive to recognize just how powerful mothers' emotions are at this time. It is so easy to place blame on your own actions and reactions and to feel that you are the source of the problem. Maintaining focus on your goal, using the knowledge and support you have amassed during your preparations for breastfeeding, and making choices that you know are in line with the lactation process and the biological aspects of breastfeeding and mothering will help you to move past these emotional binds and towards your desired outcome.

Envision what you want to have and move towards it. Keep nature in focus. Anything that is not "normal" should not be held on to. This is the time to let loose your primal being and connect with what is most natural to your biological self. Allow yourself to connect with your primal self. Accept the emotions you are feeling as a part of the experience. Don't feel bad about them; see them instead for what they are, accept them, and then let them go.

But emotions will likely play into your experience long before your new baby arrives. Having already had a difficult breastfeeding experience, you will likely find emotions surfacing that you haven't experienced since the birth of your first child. Remember that when we are not able to breastfeed, we experience a loss. If you haven't fully dealt with the emotions surrounding that loss—and let's face it, you likely haven't since at the time you had to get on with being a mother and caring for your baby—then you might need to complete the grieving process now. The typical stages of grief—denial, anger, bargaining, depression, acceptance—may not all be experienced, but it is important to realize that you will grieve the loss of your breastfeeding relationship, you might very well experience anger and depression over the loss, and in order to have the best chance of success this time around, coming to a place of acceptance is important.

Strategies you can try in order to work through lingering grief include finding support from other women who have experienced loss related to breastfeeding. Mothers Overcoming Breastfeeding Issues (MOBI) is a great place to start. MOBI maintains a website as well as a discussion list. A quick internet search will also direct you to numerous online boards discussing the issue of breastfeeding and grief. Having the support and understanding of other women, whom you do not need to convince of your grief, is important to the healing process. You might also find people around you who recognize and understand your emotions. Ask around in mothers' groups or even in your circle of friends. Too often, women do not discuss the sadness they feel when they experience breastfeeding loss and, as a result, you may not be aware that a support system is already around you. Being acknowledged and heard by your peers can help with the healing process as you move through your grief.

Try writing through your grief. Writing can be a very liberating and cathartic experience. Often, we really don't spend time recalling the actual events surrounding our experiences. Writing your memories of the experience down on paper can help you remember details you might have forgotten, focus your attention on key aspects that affected your breastfeeding efforts, such as a lack of support or a lack of information, and can give your grief shape and substance allowing you to see it for what it is and then hopefully move on from it. When we understand our experiences we can put them to better use. By writing about your experience you are likely to realize just how hard you tried to make it work. It will also likely bring back the raw emotions felt during those early days. Don't push those emotions away, but instead feel them, acknowledge them, and then promise to move on. Those emotions need not define your breastfeeding efforts. Your effort must count for something.

Acknowledge what you did do, instead of focusing on what you didn't do. Too often we look at the negative side of our actions. Okay, so in the end you were not able to breastfeed. You didn't reach your definition of breastfeeding success—or perhaps society's definition. But this doesn't negate all the honest effort you put into trying to make it work. In the six years since I published my first book, *Exclusively Pumping Breast Milk*, I have heard from hundreds and hundreds of women who were unable to breastfeed. Very rarely do I hear a story that makes me believe a mother did not do everything in her power to achieve breastfeeding success. Often I will grieve with her over the poor support she received or the failure to gain accurate information, but in almost every case, women have done everything they could to make it work given what they knew at the time or in light of the support they were given.

And you must remember that your best is largely affected by the situation you are in. It's easy to think back on your breastfeeding experience from your current position of being well-rested, confident in your parenting skills, and hormonally balanced and think that you should have been able to do more. But try to remember exactly how you were feeling at the time. When I think back to my son's first weeks of life, I get a visceral reaction. I feel overwhelmed and tense, a sense of exhaustion and frustration wells up in me, and I have an impending sense of dread. I know that at that point in my life, I *was* at the limit of what my body and my spirit could endure. Had I received a different kind of support from my family or from the professionals around me, could I have persevered further? Perhaps. But hindsight is 20/20 and when you are drowning in a rough sea of emotions being able to reach for a life ring is not always as easy as it might seem; asking for what you need can be a monumental act. Try to remember how you felt during your breastfeeding efforts, and then give yourself permission to forgive yourself.

Forgiveness is an important aspect of healing. Too often I hear from mothers who are holding on to a great deal of guilt associated with the grief they are experiencing. The biological side of breastfeeding means that we as mothers have a need to nurture our children—we crave it—and the messages of society (particularly "Breast is Best") suggest that anything less than breastfeeding is letting our children down. These forces leave so many mothers feeling a great sense of failure, guilt, and sadness—but through forgiveness you can move on. It is often easier to forgive those around us who do us wrong than it is to forgive ourselves.

And forgiving those around you is perhaps a good place to start on your healing journey. Consider those around you that provided, or should have provided, support during your early breastfeeding journey. Do you blame them or still feel anger towards them? Do you feel they let you down? Forgive them. Remember that just as you did your best at the time, these people likely were doing their best. This "best" will of course be tempered by individuals' backgrounds and knowledge and their own breastfeeding experiences. Moving forward, include these people in your breastfeeding preparations and help them improve their ability to support you.

A final aspect you may need to consider on your journey to breastfeeding your next baby is the role played by your baby. This one may be challenging. It is common for mothers to feel rejected when breastfeeding is difficult. This is a natural reaction, but it is not the reality of the situation. Babies are not rejecting their mothers when they refuse to latch. Instead, somewhere along the way the natural process—the innate reflexes and responses with which babies are born—has been disturbed. Still, mothers often feel their babies' actions are a direct reaction to them as mothers and caregivers. Laura, a mother who faced breastfeeding challenges, explains, "It took me several weeks truly to understand that there are two people in a breastfeeding relationship: no matter how much the mother desires success, how skilled she becomes, and how diligent she is, that this is only half the issue." Your baby most definitely plays an important role in breastfeeding, but he or she has no intentions or motivations with regards to his or her behaviour. Babies are purely working on instinct and reflexes.

In order to move forward into a new breastfeeding relationship, consider how you view your child in relation to the failed breastfeeding experience. Do you harbour resentment towards your child? Do you still feel that sense of rejection? Do you feel as though you must make up for what you didn't give your baby? Do you, perhaps, even blame your baby? Beginning to view breastfeeding through the biological lens may help you to resolve any challenges you are experiencing when it comes to how you view your baby's role in the breastfeeding relationship. Babies operate on instinct and reflexes. They have no understanding of why they do anything; they just do. They have a drive to survive and at times this will mean rejecting the breast. Other times this means withdrawing into a deep sleep to avoid a stressor or crying to indicate they have a need that hasn't been met.

I remember the tears I shed while attempting to nurse my son—salty tears dripping onto his little face. I felt frustrated with myself, but also with him. Why would he just not suck? Why couldn't he latch properly? Why did he prefer the bottle of expressed milk over the real deal? You can see the pattern here: Why didn't *he*... It's painful to admit, but I do think I harboured some resentment towards my son, my innocent child. Admitting this was important to my healing process. Acknowledging the frustration and resentment, seeing it for what it was, and moving on was necessary— but not easy.

Grieving is hard work. No one tells you that. Having lost both my parents within a period of four years, I now realize that grief is not something that happens; it's something you do. You must take the time to work through the emotions and the memories. Allow them to come, examine them for what they are, deal with them, and then move on. Moving on doesn't mean forgetting, but it does mean coming to a place where you can see your experience from some distance and no longer relive it every time you think of it or talk about it. The more you talk about it, the easier it will be to deal with it. The more you deal with your past breastfeeding experience, the better prepared you will be to give breastfeeding another shot, with a better chance at success.

Learning to Trust Your Body Again

As a breastfeeding mother, it can feel as though success or failure depends entirely on you. It's your body that must produce the milk to nourish your child, after all. And so what happens to your faith in your body when breastfeeding doesn't work out, when your body doesn't produce enough milk, or your anatomy seems incompatible with your baby's? In our modern society, women are given very confusing messages about our bodies. Our bodies are not acknowledged as the amazing, life-giving creations that they are, but instead as objects of beauty and desire, material to be sculpted and refined. How often are women acknowledged for their ability to birth babies or nourish infants at their breast? Rarely, if ever. So it is likely that going into motherhood you already had a lack of faith in or under-standing of your body's amazing abilities: the sheer enormity of what it means to conceive and grow a child in your womb; the power and strength necessary to birth a child into this world; or the nurturing and dedicated spirit required to nourish a baby at your breast.

When it comes to breastfeeding, our society has lost touch with the normal process and the natural interaction between mom and baby. Breastfeeding information passed between friends and family all too often uses the norms of formula feeding, which detrimentally affects normal breastfeeding. We interfere with Mother Nature's ultimate wisdom, and place our own limits and expectations onto something that in most situations should manage itself quite nicely, if everything is in balance. And through this societal interference in the breastfeed-ing relationship, mothers have lost faith in their bodies' ability to produce milk and nourish babies.

This loss of faith, though, is initiated long before our babies' births. Throughout pregnancy we are given messages that suggest our bodies are not capable of childbirth and that we must rely on medicine and men to help us birth our babies. Your doctor might talk to you about pain management during labour or the possible interventions that may be needed. Sometimes pregnant women will be given labour timelines which, if they don't or can't follow, will lead to the implementation of other, more aggressive measures. It is common for women to be told that if they labour for x number of hours without any progres-sion, they will need to use pitocin or if they go x number of days past their due date an induction will need to be carried out. Somehow we as women have been convinced that our bodies must follow the schedule that medicine dictates, instead of medicine following the natural schedule of our bodies.

If we are made to believe our bodies are incapable of birthing our babies, and inductions and c-sections are necessary in record numbers in order to bring our children into this world, is it any wonder that women are also convinced that this insufficiency also extends to our efforts to nourish our babies? But part of the process of overcoming a difficult breastfeeding experience is recognizing the power you have as a woman, the power of your body to not only birth your babies but also nourish your babies, and reclaiming the strengths and power that makes you a woman.

Now I realize that this may all sound a little like flower child, crunchy granola, new-age thinking, but if we truly believe that breastfeeding is the biologically normal method of feeding and something worth striving for, then we must also accept the biological nature of our bodies and the ability we have to follow through with this biological process. So how do we do this? How do we make this shift in thinking? How do we reconnect to that which makes us women? A good place to start is to educate ourselves and understand where our modern society has gone wrong—what has thrown us off track.

Earlier in the book we discussed many of the societal influences on breastfeeding. The impact of modern medicine has also been investigated. It is important to recognize that very rarely is it our bodies that fail us, but instead it is society and the medical system that negatively affect normal breastfeeding. Consider your past breastfeeding experience in the light of this information. Actually get out a piece of paper and create two columns: one column titled society and one titled medicine. Go through your own labour and breastfeeding story and begin filling in the columns. If you are like most women, it won't take you long to create a substantial list. Now consider your own body: is there blame to place there?

Most likely, your body is the one thing that didn't fail you. Your body did what it was supposed to do, and when confronted with medical procedures that affected lactation or societal influences that were counter to breastfeeding success, it did the best it could. And now with new information, and a better understanding of the aspects of society and medicine that might affect breastfeeding, you can help your body do what it is meant to do. Be empowered by a renewed sense of purpose and knowledge. You have the ability to guard against the forces that work counter to successful lactation. Your body is meant to nourish your child.

It can be a leap of faith to trust in your body again. I understand that completely. After my body developed preeclampsia, I felt very strongly that I—that my body—had let my son down. It took a lot of reflecting and a lot of time to get myself to a place where I believed my body could successfully carry a baby to term, birth a child, and nourish a child. I worried throughout my second pregnancy that it would fail again, but each day was a bit easier, and I realized that my worry only gave power to society and the medical establishment. I had to take the power back. Whatever the outcome, I needed to go into the experience believing that my body was capable and that I would limit the negative effect from outside sources in order to give my body a fighting chance.

And fight you may have to. This can be a difficult battle to overcome. Believing we *can't* becomes a self-fulfilling prophecy; if we believe we can't, we often make it so. Sharon experienced this doubt, sharing, "I was not as confident because of the previous difficulties I had. Now looking back, a lot of it was probably just normal 'getting to know your baby' kind of difficulty." It can be easy to psyche yourself out, so you must actively work to empower yourself. Remember your goal, define your success, don't develop expectations, but instead be ready to participate in the experience and make choices based on your sound knowledge of the biological nature of breastfeeding. The end result is very much worth it.

Regaining that trust in your body is liberating. Making breastfeeding work the second time around helps to heal many of the hurts and pains from the first experience. In *Unbuttoned*, Heidi Raykeil explains, "Breastfeeding my daughter taught me to trust my body again, to feel safe in the world, to count on something and have somebody count on me...It sustained me, and it tethered me with a safe, predictable connection to the most important thing in the world."[2] This is what we aim for and hope for. While there are no guarantees in this world, learning to trust your body, and the power it holds, will go a long way to healing the loss of your first breastfeeding experience.

Arm Yourself with Information

Information is critical to success. Once upon a time, breastfeeding knowledge was passed along from generation to generation. A young girl would learn about baby care and breastfeeding by watching her mother, her sisters, her aunts, and her friends. It was a fact of life and a way of life. Now that implicit knowledge has been lost. We are forced to educate ourselves; in order to give yourself the best possible chance at a positive breastfeeding experience, you must seek out evidence-based information that approaches breastfeeding from a biological, rather than societal, perspective.

Information can be gathered from numerous types of sources: books, DVDs, classes, the internet, and support groups. I encourage you to seek out all of these. But as you search for information, be prepared to assess its value. Consider the perspective from which it is approaching breastfeeding. Is it glossing over the important biological aspects and dealing more with scheduling, timing, positioning, and sleeping? Or is it focusing on the biological nature of breastfeeding: the process of lactation and how it affects breastfeeding management, the needs of a baby and how breastfeeding meets those needs, and the ways in which a mother and her support system can understand and respond to the innate needs of a baby while still managing life? You need to become adept at assessing the information being presented to you. There are some excellent resources out there, and there are some absolutely horrible resources that jeopardize breastfeeding instead of supporting it.

As previously mentioned, consider the importance of breast-feeding and then compare that with the length of time usually devoted to it in a pre-natal class. I encourage you to try to locate a class that is solely focused on breastfeeding as opposed to a prenatal class in which breastfeeding is merely a short portion. Seek out classes taught by qualified breastfeeding specialists such as an International Board Certified Lactation Consultant (IBCLC).[3] Contact your local midwifery group or chapter of La Leche League to connect with classes that might fit your needs.

La Leche League and other such breastfeeding support groups are also good places to find other women who have practical experience and who may provide positive assistance with your new baby. Your local health unit may have breastfeed-ing support. Perhaps even your hospital offers an out-patient breastfeeding support group. Ask around and begin to build a list of resources and sources of information — information that you can access both during your pregnancy and after the birth of your child. Keep the information accessible and tell your spouse where the information is located. If you do experience difficulties with your new baby, you don't want to have to do a lot of work to find the information you need.

Breastfeeding information on the internet is easily accessible, always available, and often anonymous. This anonymity may be attractive to some people. For Charlotte, taking a breastfeeding class during her second pregnancy, after having a difficult time breastfeeding her first baby, was not something she was comfortable doing. She explains, "I didn't take any classes before the birth of my second because I felt like I would be judged for what happened with my daughter and I also felt that the challenges we faced were not normal and that nobody would be able to help or understand."

The anonymity of the internet can be a great thing, but it can also be a negative. You never truly know from whom the information is coming. Even formula companies will provide breastfeeding information. How reliable can it be? How much of an interest do they really have in a mom's breastfeeding success? If using information from the internet, consider the source very carefully. Websites such as Kellymom.com, La Leche League, or Dr. Jack Newman's site provide sound, evidence-based information. Many breastfeeding support organizations also have online support. There are numerous national organizations that will provide individual support via telephone or email. Again, make it a point during your pregnancy to locate and access these sources of information. Bookmark them. Have the toll free numbers written down and posted in a prominent place.

Social networking is a big part of today's connected world. Don't overlook this as a potential source of support and information. Online social networks such as Facebook provide many opportunities to connect with other mothers, organizations, and information sources. As always, you need to assess the merits of each and judge the information and support they are providing against your knowledge, but once you find a network of support it can prove to be invaluable.

Organize a Support System

Moving outwards from the core which is the mother-baby relationship, the support you have around you can make an enormous difference to breastfeeding success and longevity. Creating a support system during your pregnancy can be a way of healing the residual hurt from your past breastfeeding experience and can give you a sense of strength knowing that there is a large circle of family and friends working with you to create a strong breastfeeding relationship between you and your new baby. Heather reflects on the importance of this support saying, "Once I started to investigate other mothers' stories I started to feel better about myself, my son, and our situation." Support can come from those closest to you, from groups created for the purpose of support, or from very unexpected places. I remember having an older man comment on how lovely it was to see a baby nursing and what a wonderful thing I was doing for my daughter. A simple acknowledgement such as this can go a long way to encourage you in difficult times.

Pregnancy is the time to consider your support system. It is the time to look honestly at your family and friends and determine if anyone may not be completely supportive of your goals. It's not enough for you to have the goal. If you have a family member who is quick to suggest you feed formula every time your baby has difficulties latching, for example, this undermines your confidence and puts negativity into the air. The immediate post-partum period is not the time to have to deal with meddling parents or overbearing friends. Make your needs and intentions clear to anyone you feel may not be on board with your plans to breastfeed. Explain to them the importance of it for you and what it is you need from them. And then enlist the help of your spouse or partner to ensure compliance after the birth of your baby.

Just as you should never have to fight to get the birth experience you want, you shouldn't have to fight to get the support you need once your baby arrives. Have a person designated to fight these fights for you. An obvious choice is your partner. This is an important role for fathers. Fathers are the protectors of both mom and baby. They have the crucial role of ensuring balance is maintained in the home, no distractions or threats present themselves, and that mom and baby can get on with the business of bonding and establishing their breastfeeding relationship. Make sure your partner is very clear on the importance of breastfeeding to you; including him in your process of breast-feeding education is a great way to help him understand the biological aspects of breastfeeding and the ways he can help support you. Dads should also come to any appointments you might have with lactation consultants since they can help you remember the information given and remind you of key pieces of knowledge at appropriate times. The father should be given every power necessary, including asking guests to leave if they are not willing to support your efforts. Limiting visiting times to those periods where you have your partner for support is also a good strategy if you are concerned about the way visitors will try to influence your breastfeeding relationship.

As you progress through your pregnancy, begin to establish a list of support people. Who do you know who has breastfed their baby? What local groups provide breastfeeding support? Is your doctor breastfeeding friendly? Do you know of any lactation consultants in your area? (If not, find one and consider meeting with her prior to the birth of your baby.) What friends can you call on when you are having a hard time and need to talk to someone? Who might be willing to come by for a while and help with housework or the care of a younger child when you need a break? Make a list and again, display it prominently so you have access to it when you need it.

It is important to note that support doesn't always have to be breastfeeding support. Although breastfeeding may be at the top of the list—and is the subject of this book—other types of support are important. If you have a younger child running around the house, having someone who can provide occasional childcare would be a blessing. Laundry, housework, cooking: all these things can quickly overburden a new mother. Consider all these needs when building a support network.

Another possibility might be to hire a doula. Doulas are often thought of as women who attend your birth and support you and your partner through the process. But doulas also work with new moms after a baby's birth. A doula can provide instruction on baby care, assist with common tasks such as bathing, provide breastfeeding assistance, and some may even offer light house-keeping or childcare for older children. While there is an expense involved hiring a doula, the cost may very well be worth it if she is able to help you achieve your breastfeeding goals. To locate a doula or post-partum doula in your area, contact one of the organizations that certify doula such as Childbirth International or DONA International.

Check Your Expectations

We all have expectations. Perhaps it's part of the human condi-tion to create plans and expectations for the future and for experiences to come. But when reality and expectations do not match up, we are often left feeling disappointed and potentially feeling as though we lost something, failed, or were cheated out of something that was already ours. What are your expectations for labour and delivery, motherhood, parenting, and marriage once your new baby arrives, and how do they fit with normal breastfeeding?

What is biologically normal is always central to the successful experience of breastfeeding. When you fight against nature, it can create severe difficulties. It is well worth your time and effort, prior to having another baby, to seek out information and think back to your first baby in order to figure out what are normal expectations—biologically speaking—and what are not.

Do you expect your baby to sleep through the night at four weeks of age? This is not biologically expected behaviour. Do you expect your baby to calmly hang out in a bassinet while you make dinner? Not likely and not biologically expected. Do you expect that you will be able to sleep for eight hours after delivery and then breastfeed your baby for the first time? Again, not the ideal as far as biological expectations go. Do you expect your two month-old to nurse only four or five times a day, tanking up like a formula-fed baby might with 8 oz. bottles? This isn't going to happen. Understanding what is biologically expected can help us to frame and evaluate our own expectations and how they may or may not be met. Understanding biological expectations can also show us how our own misguided expectations can interfere with successful breastfeeding.

Time to sleep or to spend with your spouse or a natural delivery without medications may all be desirable to you, but it's important to differentiate between what you would *like* to happen and what you *expect* to happen. Rarely in life do things go exactly as we hope. Things happen. It's a fact of life. When preparing for your next child and breastfeeding experience, educate yourself as much as you can. This knowledge will serve you well when you are confronted with situations that don't fit into your expected or desired outcome. For example, if your baby is born prematurely, you will know from your newly gained information that early stimulation is critical to establishing a good milk supply and that if you can't nurse your baby right away, you will need to start pumping as soon as possible and as frequently as possible, just as a newborn would be nursing. By informing yourself, making decisions, and taking action based on your knowledge, you will guide your experience. The outcome isn't always in our power to control, but the way we react to our experience is. Making these decisions based on the experience you find yourself in instead of on expectations you might have is important not only for decisions that you might personally need to implement, but also for those working with and caring for you. While every doctor undoubtedly wants a healthy baby, not all doctors are knowledgeable about breast-feeding and their recommendations may interfere with a success-ful breastfeeding outcome. Don't hesitate to ask questions and request alternatives in your care and your baby's care.

It is not enough to expect to breastfeed, you must make the choices and create the experience that will allow that outcome. The steps to breastfeeding may very well not be what you imagine them to be, but by taking an active role in your experi-ence and making choices based on your knowledge of normal breastfeeding, you can help direct yourself to your ultimate goal.

It's a Process

Prior to having your first child, did you think about the wonders of motherhood? Did you consider the complexity and sheer miracle of the entire process and experience? If you are like most women, the sheer enormity of the experience completely blind-sided you. Our society just doesn't do motherhood justice. And you were likely caught off-guard when you realized that the emotions you had for this new, little creature in your arms were overwhelming and completely out of your control. Becoming a mother is a powerful experience.

There is an amazing bond between a mother and her child devised most certainly by a higher power. Mother Nature, God—whatever you choose to call this power—has devised a way to have mothers and children so closely linked that it can cause physical pain when we are separated. This close connec-tion is truly awe-inspiring. However, in spite of the power of this natural bond, when we interfere with the normal processes of bonding and attachment we can also affect the normal outcomes.

The normal process of motherhood and lactation, the biological aspects of breastfeeding, and the hormonal aspects of breastfeeding and bonding have all been discussed previously in this book. They are all important areas to research and consider as you prepare for the arrival of your next baby. The overriding thesis of this book is that breastfeeding is a biologically expected and normal process and in order to have the best chance of establishing a successful breastfeeding relationship, this biological process needs to be respected and protected.

So how do you view motherhood? How do you view breastfeeding? How do you view bonding?

There is no one right answer here, but take some time as you plan for your new baby's arrival to really ponder these questions. If you are like me, and I suspect most women in our society, your ideas of motherhood and breastfeeding will be tangled up with false information and beliefs more closely related to the norms of formula feeding. Your ideas might be tied to how you perceive yourself as a woman and the value placed on a woman's role in society. Childhood experiences can also shape our views on mothering and breastfeeding as with Michelle who, from a young age, felt there were "two distinct categories" of women: "those who are the 'type to breastfeed' and those who are not" and who firmly placed herself in the latter category. We come into motherhood with a lot of baggage—and notions about what motherhood will be like. These notions can sometimes surprise us by actually coming true; but more often we are quickly brought back to reality when we realize that things aren't as we were led to believe or as we ourselves wanted to believe.

Think about your preparations as a journey. We all come to motherhood from different places. As clichéd as the phrase may be, we may truly find the journey to be just as important as the destination. Learning to connect with our true selves can be a great reward. By considering who we are as women and mothers and how those roles are influenced by our biological natures, and learning to trust in the innate abilities we have instead of fighting them, motherhood—and, if I may say, even womanhood—can be a much more fulfilling experience.

Denying our biological nature, especially when it comes to childbirth, breastfeeding, and mothering, can have serious consequences. If we desire the biologically expected outcome—the breastfeeding relationship—we can't ignore the biological process. As you consider breastfeeding your next child, spend some time thinking about how the outcome is supported by the process and what that means for you as a mother.

New Approaches (or a return to the old)

I have stated from the beginning that I am not presenting a "how-to" book on breastfeeding. There are plenty of those already on the market and many of them do a much better job than I could of presenting current, evidence-based information in an easily accessible format. I do, however, want to just briefly introduce the work of two women, Suzanne Colson and Christina Smillie, who are offering something new in the world of breastfeeding. In reality, their ideas are old and are a return to knowledge and understanding about breastfeeding that has been lost to us over the generations. The ideas presented by these women are based on the importance of the biological process of breastfeeding and respect the knowledge and skills inherent to both mothers and babies.

Biological Nurturing—Suzanne Colson

The subtitle of Suzanne Colson's website is "laid back breastfeeding" and Colson's work and ideas are based on that idea in both a literal and figurative sense. Breastfeeding should most definitely be "laid back" in the sense that it shouldn't be stressful and should seamlessly fit into your daily life. Breastfeeding positions can also be laid back, both in attitude and practice.

Colson describes biological nurturing (BN) in this way:

> BN is laid back breastfeeding: mothers neither sit upright nor do they lie on their sides or flat on their backs. Instead, they are in comfortable semi-reclined positions where every part of their body is supported especially their shoulders and neck. Then they lay their babies on top of their bodies so that baby's head is somewhere near the breast. In other words mothers make the breast available. Babies lie prone or on their tummies but their bodies are not flat but tilted up.[4]

On her website, Biological Nurturing, Colson presents these basic beliefs about breastfeeding:

- Mothers and babies are versatile feeders. There is not one way to breastfeed.
- A baby does not need to be awake to latch on and feed.
- Babies often self-attach; mothers can help them do this.
- Babies often have reflex movements called cues indicating they are ready to feed whilst asleep.
- Looking for baby reflex feeding cues helps mothers to get to know their babies sooner. This increases confidence.
- Crying and hunger cues are late feeding indicators often making latching difficult. Getting started with breastfeeding is about releasing baby feeding reflexes as stimulants, helping ba-

bies find the breast, latch on and feed... not about interest.

- The breastfeeding position the baby uses often mimics the baby in the womb.
- There is no right or wrong breastfeeding position. The right position is the one that works.
- Babies do not always feed for hunger; "non nutritive sucking" is hugely beneficial to increase your milk and satisfy your baby's needs.[5]

Breastfeeding should be a time of relaxation for both mom and baby, but all too often new mothers are stressed and anxious about breastfeeding their newborns. Breastfeeding supporters often show new moms very specific breastfeeding positions or even physically handle mom and baby to try to force a latch. Having had this experience myself when my son was still in the NICU, I know how humiliating and stressful this can be, and I've heard from many women who have had similar experiences and talk of how violated and uncomfortable they felt with such aggressive breastfeeding support.

Suzanne Colson approaches breastfeeding from a perspective of calm and relaxation. Not only is this the approach for the actual act of breastfeeding, but for the way that breastfeeding fits into your life. Breastfeeding should be easy; it should fit easily into your life. While it is true that many women today have life situations that take them outside of the home during the day and do not allow for full-time breastfeeding, even when this is the case, breastfeeding when you are with your child can be an easy, stress-reducing way of mothering, bonding with, and nurturing your baby.

I strongly encourage you to visit Suzanne Colson's website, www.biologicalnurturing.com, and learn more about her ideas and suggestions for breastfeeding. Her article, "A non-prescriptive recipe for breastfeeding", available on her website, is a great introduction to the idea of biological nurturing. She has also recently published a book called *An Introduction to Biological Nurturing.* If you have an interest in using the method with your next baby, you might consider purchasing a copy or asking for it at your local library.

Baby-led Latching—Christina Smillie

If indeed birth and breastfeeding are biological processes, is it any wonder that babies are born with a unique and amazing set of skills and reflexes that facilitate their ability to breastfeed? Christina Smillie has extensively researched newborns' breast-feeding abilities and her approach, based on this research, is commonly referred to as baby-led latching. Dr. Smillie recognizes that babies have a sequence of behaviours that lead them to latching. When this sequence is followed, latching becomes easier and less stressful for both mom and baby.

Babies are born with reflexes that assist them in breastfeeding. These reflexes include:

- Stepping and crawling, which help a baby get to the breast.
- Searching, rooting, sight, and smell, which help a baby find the breast.
- Rooting and opening the mouth, helping a baby attach to the breast.
- Sucking, which is stimulated when a baby feels the nipple in the mouth.

Skin-to-skin contact on the mother's chest stimulates a baby's sense of smell and touch, which initiates feeding behaviours. A calm, attentive state—for both mother and baby—assists in feeding behaviours and helps the newborn find the breast and successfully breastfeed. It is important to find a position in which you are comfortable (just as Suzanne Colson suggests). A relaxed mom is just as important as a relaxed baby.

The following is a brief overview of baby-led latching:

- Place baby in a vertical position between your breasts, skin-to-skin. Your baby can be in a diaper. You should be in a somewhat reclined position.
- Support your baby's neck and shoulders but not the head. A baby has a reflex to push back on anything holding its head.
- Support your baby's bottom as well. You can use the crook of your arm to support your baby's rump and legs. Your baby needs to feel safe and secure.
- Follow your baby's lead: if baby wants to sleep, sleep is okay. Allow your baby to set the pace. Your job is to keep your baby calm.
- When your baby gets hungry, she will start to search for the breast by bobbing her head around. Support the baby's neck and shoulders as the baby moves towards the breast but allow free head movement.
- Support your baby's bottom with the other hand and keep your baby's tummy tight to your chest. Do not allow the legs to flail around. Help your baby feel secure.
- If necessary, help your baby line up with the nipple: nose to nipple and chin in close contact with the breast. Your baby will likely nuzzle, lick,

and taste before actually latching. Be patient and allow your baby to figure it all out.

- Calm and talk to your baby throughout. If your baby is anxious, soothe him by talking gently or making *shhhhing* sounds. If necessary, you may need to remove your baby from your chest and swaddle and soothe him before returning him skin-to-skin.

- Do not try to force your baby to the breast. Only offer the breast when your baby is calm. Pay attention to early feeding cues and keep your newborn skin-to-skin as much as possible to allow frequent feeding at the baby's pace.

- If your baby has had difficulty establishing breastfeeding or has refused to latch, baby-led latching can be a gentle way to encourage breastfeeding.[6]

There is a significant amount of information on the internet about baby-led latching including numerous videos. What is most important with this approach is the respect for the biological process and the understanding that babies are born with a great many skills to assist them to breastfeed successfully. Listening to our babies and allowing them to follow their own instincts can go a long way to establishing a strong breastfeeding relationship.

These are just two different sources that you may not otherwise come across, but which contain information returning breastfeeding to a more normal, biological process. Both Suzanne Colson and Christina Smillie recognize the important of listening to our babies and following the sage advice of Mother Nature.

This chapter has looked at many different elements that combine to assist in establishing a successful breastfeeding relationship, including the idea of what success actually is. Ultimately, the experience is yours, regardless of what the outcome may be. It is important to embrace your breastfeeding experience, both past and future, and claim it as your own. Even if you only breastfed your first time around for a couple of weeks, you did breastfeed. Every mother and baby eventually wean, some just earlier than others. Rather than always providing the disclaimer in your answer to the question "did you breastfeed?" learn to say, "yes, I did." While it might not have been the experience you expected or hoped for, it has brought you to where you are today, and I would strongly suggest that it has made you a better, more empathetic person, capable of far more than you ever once thought possible.

Head into your new breastfeeding experience feeling empowered and strong. You will come out the other side a different person than when you started. Stay focused on your goal, but recognize the power and importance of the journey itself.

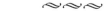

Heather's Story

The minute I found out I was expecting my first child back in 2005 I knew right then and there that I was going to breastfeed and give them the best start in life I could. I did my research, asked questions of friends and experts, bought all the required supplies (breast pads, storage bottles, pump, breastfeeding-friendly bottles, etc.). I was *ready* and *willing*. This was something that was going to come naturally!

My pregnancy was pretty routine up until thirty-eight weeks when I developed pregnancy-induced hypertension that was borderline preeclampsia. My water broke at exactly thirty-nine weeks and I was admitted to labour and delivery and induced immediately—all of a sudden I was slapped in the face by reality—this was not part of my birth plan and things were not going the way I had envisioned them.

After twenty-one straight hours of an induction, I failed to progress and an emergency c-section was forced upon me. When I returned to my room for the first time after recovery, I either had a nurse saying, "You must breastfeed right now!" or me telling myself, *I have to feed my child right at this moment!* Now remember I *wanted* to breastfeed. I was prepared...but what I was not prepared for was the lack of sleep (up for close to thirty-six hours), sheer exhaustion, and post-op recovery from major surgery. My intentions were grand but my will was shattered. So I decided to sleep and to give it 100% in the morning—a new day, a new beginning!

Approximately six hours after I had delivered (the following morning), I decided it was time: time to feed my baby, my child. I had a wonderful nursing staff that was eager and very willing to help me step-by-step in the process. I was shown various holds, provided with tips and tricks, and away I went. My son was on my breast and latching like a true champ—like he knew this was something we had both agreed to take on and accomplish together—our first true bonding experience as mother and son. We did this time and time again, every few hours. I thought after our first few feedings, *Wow, this is amazing! What a wonderful experience.*

However, after a few days in, I realized things are not always as they seem. Call it mother's intuition, but I started to pick up on signs that perhaps this wasn't going as well as I thought it was. My son was still fighting the jaundice he was born with; he seemed irritable and what I guess I would call hungry. I started to get a sinking and panicky feeling that he wasn't actually getting anything—was I not keeping up my end of the bargain?

I asked the nurse if I could pump to see if I could possibly build up a supply and maybe try feeding by a different method. They agreed, and I was hooked up to the double milking machine (really, if you haven't tried this wild contraption, you haven't lived)! I was hooked up in front of, and to the delight of, my husband and mother. It was a little awkward to say the least, but I was determined to feed my child.

It didn't take long on the "milker" to realize the root of my problem. The wonderful golden drink of the gods, colostrum, that is supposed to be the key to providing your baby with the essential needs right after birth, was absent from my body—there was nothing there. I was devastated and that night when I was alone, I broke down. Why could I not do the thing I wanted to do most for my child? Why?

The next day the nurses kept trying to encourage me to put my baby to my breast but I was getting frustrated quickly. I had mixed emotions and the fact that my child was not getting any nourishment was weighing heavily on my mind. I was introduced to the Supplemental Nursing System and tried to feed my little one formula via the tiny tube taped to my breast. He did suck and was getting some formula but the process was upsetting and the tape kept coming off. It ended up being more of a nightmare and continued to add to my frustration. I was then introduced to finger feeding with the SNS but was not successful. My son would not take it and this again made both of us more and more frustrated.

Finally on the fourth day in the hospital and after numerous hours of trying to feed my son, I broke down completely. I asked for formula and a bottle. I needed to get him something to eat. They reluctantly agreed (this again frustrated me more) and their reluctance only added to my mounting guilt at not being able to provide for my child. That was the day we were to leave the hospital and go out into the world on our own; I was still determined to win the breastfeeding battle. My son had lost 9% of his body weight in the four days since his birth and they allowed us to leave—granted he was now eating like a champ on the bottle-fed formula.

On my way home I stopped and bought a medical grade pump, as I was as determined as ever to breastfeed my child; I still had confidence I could do this. I figured that in the comfort of my own home, under my own routine, I could adjust to my little one and we could find a rhythm of our own.

So I tried for six days—pumping, putting baby to my breast, and supplementing with the bottle-fed formula; he was latching fine but I was still unable to provide him with any sustenance. It was within those six days that my son decided on his own that he preferred the bottle. Soon he would wince at the sight of my breast coming to his mouth and would turn away, fussing. I knew right then and there the bottle had won! Really, I cannot blame him. It was like I was teasing him to suck on a nipple that would not deliver. That night and for a few nights after I wallowed in my guilt—I had failed—why, how could this have happened? Where was my milk?

Lo and behold, on the eleventh day of trying my milk came in with a vengeance. I was in the shower that morning and it started to pour—like two fountains. I was overwhelmed with excitement! I once again tried to put my son to my breast but he wanted nothing of it. Again, I felt discouraged, guilty and defeated. Why had it taken so long for my milk to come in? And, now that I had it, why would he not take it? So just as I had done my research on breastfeeding, I started my research on milk production and rejecting the breast. What I learned in this journey was that I should *not* feel guilty. I did what I could and nature was against me.

I realized I had many factors that were stacked against me and all of these combined came into play to defeat me. I had delivered early and via a section and had possibly not released the timely hormones which tell the body to start producing milk. Apparently this can happen as a result of c-section. Once I started to investigate other mothers' stories I started to feel better about myself, my son, and our situation. My guilt started to fade and I realized I had tried; tried the best I could and gave it my all. Looking back now, I may have given up a little too easily — why did I not pump once my milk came in and take advantage of the ample milk supply? I think I had my reasons at the time.

Now, four years later I am once again blessed with another chance, another shot to give it my all with breastfeeding. I am expecting my second child and I have not wavered in my intentions. I am going into this experience again with the same faith and vigour as I did the first time; however, this time I am much wiser, more experienced, and more educated. This time I have more ideas and back-up plans. I plan on trying again straight to the breast but know I will be faced with possible issues as I will be delivering via c-section again. However, this time I am in control. I know it is coming. I will know the date and time and be prepared!

I will not harbour the same guilt if things do not work out the way I want them to, but I know it will not mean I have failed! I am planning to pump should the baby not take to the breast, and I plan on doing this for as long as I can to provide my newest child with the start that I could not provide my first! I know there will be challenges along the way but my eyes are opened wider. I know I will succeed this time around but in what form? Well, time will tell.

I encourage all mothers to try; there is nothing lost if you at least try. And I want to let mothers know that if they don't want to try for your own reasons, that is fine too. As mothers we know what is right for our children. This guilt for not breastfeeding shouldn't be there! My first-born (now 4) has turned out to be a healthy vibrant little man who sets out each and every day to conquer the world, and yes, he was formula-fed! I go into motherhood a second time with a new outlook and relish the second chance I have been given!

An Update from Heather—Ten Months Later

The birth of my second baby came after a wonderful ten months of pregnancy, although almost four years after the first. The only issue I had was the dreaded morning sickness. My blood pressure stayed down, no preeclampsia symptoms, and I pushed for a VBAC (vaginal birth after c-section)! I was sent for a bio-physical at forty-one weeks and everything showed things were fine with the baby, so I was allowed to continue to forty-one weeks five days at which time my provider was willing to perform a mild induction to get the ball rolling, even though it would put me into a higher risk zone for uterine rupture. However, my health history during the pregnancy was favour-able.

Then with the induction looming in two days, I went into spontaneous labour. After a very productive thirteen-hour labour I gave birth on my own to a beautiful 9lbs. 3oz. baby boy—twenty minutes, ten pushes and not a rip, tear or stitch to write home about! It was such a natural high. I have never felt anything like it before. I could have pushed ten babies out. I was so elated!

So, as you can see, pregnancies and births from one child to another—night and day!

As for the breastfeeding, this too followed suit. The major issues from the first time came so naturally the second time around. From about nineteen weeks onward I had colostrum and was leaking from time to time. Only a few hours after my second son was born I had him on the breast and his latch and suck were fantastic—it was like we both had a job to do and something to prove! Again, I was elated—I could provide for my baby! It was what I wanted so badly for my first but could not do!

Now, it wasn't all roses. Brigham was jaundiced and had to spend some time in phototherapy, so feeding was a challenge with him being so sleepy. I did supplement from days three to five but always put him to the breast before and after the bottle-feedings. On about day four my milk came in and we had a night of hell where he was so hungry and I was so engorged that it made both of us crazy. Luckily I had one can of formula on hand so that got us through the night!

About a week after his birth he was nursing like a champ. He feeds very well, and we have fallen into a nice little routine now at two months. I weighed him the other day and he is already up to fifteen pounds, so I would say he is doing just fine and getting plenty to eat! I feel so proud of both of us!

I love watching him eat. I love his expressions at the breast. I love his drunk little look when he comes off and just that close connection we have together. It is everything I thought it would be and more! My plan was to make it six months breastfeeding, but now two months in, I can see this being a lot longer relation-ship than I ever expected.

I guess what I would tell other moms who have had issues in the past or feel defeated is to just give it another chance. There are many factors I believe defeated me the first time around, and I think the stars were aligned this time and I was even more determined to make it work!

Breastfeeding, Take Two

And If It Should Happen Again?

"In the long term, I think it taught me that motherhood isn't about being perfect...I wonder if I got too consumed in using my ability to provide breast milk to prove my worthiness as a mother."

Sharon, mom of two

Even with the best intentions and preparation, it is possible that breastfeeding may prove difficult the second time around. But it is my hope that through the information provided in this book, you will have formed a new attitude about breastfeeding and gained an understanding of why it is such an important aspect of the mother-baby relationship—and as such you will also understand how you can enjoy a satisfying relationship with your baby, even if you are not able to achieve your ideal breastfeeding experience.

Determining Your Own Success

Throwing out the expectations of society and really reaching inside yourself as a mother can help you to establish your own success. What do *you* really want and how can you achieve it? What does it mean to be a mother? Is it defined by how you feed your child? It is true that breastfeeding allows for a different bonding experience than does bottle-feeding; but it is just that— different. While it is the biologically normal means of bonding, if you don't achieve it, all hope is not lost. Bonding through

229

breastfeeding is only one means of establishing a strong relationship with your child. Your value as a mother cannot be determined by the method by which you feed your child. Likewise, your success as a mother is not determined by whether or not you are able to breastfeed.

Breastfeeding is one aspect of mothering; it is not the only aspect. What other activities, responsibilities, and actions are part of mothering in your mind? Focus on what you do have, instead of what you might not have. Consider all the things you do for your child, all the ways you nurture and nourish your child. Give yourself credit where it is due. Determine your own success. Too often, we view our failures as though they are what define us. Make a conscious effort to use your successes to define yourself. As mothers, we will always have things that we could do better, but focusing on what we are doing well can help us keep moving forward and struggling through the challenges that motherhood also brings. Should breastfeeding the second time around bring with it challenges, and perhaps ultimately not work out, focus not on the loss but the success.

Nurturing Your Baby in Other Ways

Breastfeeding is not only a method of providing nutrition for a baby but also a way of nurturing. You can nurture your baby as a breastfeeding mother does even if you do not nourish your baby at the breast. Breastfeeding provides closeness, responsiveness, and control to babies. As a mother who is bottle-feeding, these qualities of breastfeeding can be implemented allowing you and your baby a close relationship through the feeding experience. The following is a partial list of some of the ways you can include aspects of breastfeeding even when breastfeeding itself doesn't work out. These are not exhaustive, nor are they prescriptive. You can choose to use just one, or you may want to incorporate all of the ideas into your parenting practice.

Paced Bottle-feeding

Paced bottle-feeding, sometimes referred to as bottle-nursing, is a means of bottle-feeding that more closely follows normal breastfeeding behaviours. Breastfeeding provides a great deal of interaction between mom and baby and also provides baby a great deal of control over how often to nurse and how much milk baby drinks. Some of the keys to paced bottle-feeding include:

- Allow the baby to draw the bottle nipple into his or her mouth instead of forcing or placing the nipple into the mouth.
- Feed according to normal, early feeding cues as opposed to feeding on a schedule.
- Hold the bottle in a horizontal position. Tilt it vertically only enough to keep milk in the nipple.
- Hold the baby in an upright position. Do not re-cline the baby during feeding.
- Switch sides during the feeding session.
- Pace the feeding so that it lasts 10-20 minutes. Do not allow your baby to guzzle the bottle.
- Take frequent breaks during the feeding session. Just as a nursing baby has periods of active nursing and rest, a bottle-feed baby will benefit from frequent breaks when feeding. Rest the bottle nipple on the baby's chin or cheek during the break and then allow the baby to draw the nipple back into his or her mouth when ready to resume feeding.
- Allow the baby to indicate fullness. Do not encourage a baby to finish a bottle.[1]

Paced bottle-feeding should, ideally, be practiced by anyone bottle-feeding any baby.

Proximity

There are many ways that you can ensure close proximity with your baby, regardless of whether you are breastfeeding or not. When you are not breastfeeding, proximity is important to provide the close contact that babies (and let's face it, mothers too) crave. Close proximity can be encouraged through skin-to-skin time, co-sleeping or close proximity sleeping, and baby-wearing. You might choose to use some or all of these in order to share a close physical connection with your baby.

Skin-to-skin time is a wonderful way to bond with your newborn. It can be a very effective means of establishing breastfeeding, but even when breastfeeding is no longer in the picture, spending time skin-to-skin with your baby can provide wonderful closeness and an opportunity to get to know your baby. You can practice skin-to-skin time in many different ways, but the key aspect is simply the skin-to-skin contact between mom and baby. Undress your baby down to the diaper and place your baby on your bare chest, then lay back and relax, enjoying the connection with your little one.

Co-sleeping has been practiced since the beginning of time. It does, however, need to be done safely and with precautions taken. If you decide that co-sleeping is something that you would like to do, it is important to take the following into consideration:

- Do not sleep with your baby if you, or your partner, smoke or have taken any drugs—prescription, non-prescription, or illicit—or are under the influence of alcohol.
- Ensure all bedding fits tightly on the mattress and that there are no fluffy duvets or loose blankets around your baby's face.

- Ensure your mattress fits tightly against the headboard.
- Ensure there are no gaps between the wall and mattress in which the baby can get trapped.
- Do not place your baby on her stomach to sleep.
- If your spouse is uncomfortable with the baby in bed with you, consider other arrangements.
- If you or your spouse have a history of deep sleep, sleep apnea, sleep walking, or any sleep disorders, consider other alternatives.
- Do not sleep with your baby if you or your partner are considered medically obese.
- Do not allow other children or pets onto the bed while co-sleeping.

Co-sleeping is not the only arrangement that will provide close proximity between you and your baby. You might also consider placing your baby's crib in your bedroom, which will allow you to hear and sense your baby during the night. Side-car type cribs and bassinets that attach to the side of your bed are also available, allowing you to attend to your baby easily during the night while avoiding some of the potential dangers of co-sleeping.

Babywearing is simply the use of a baby carrier to facilitate carrying your baby. You can wear your baby from birth until a couple of years of age and beyond. Finding a carrier that you are comfortable using and one that safely supports your baby can be a freeing experience. Baby carriers free up your hands, allowing you to carry on with daily activities and interests, while at the same time providing your baby with the closeness they desire and direct interaction with you and the world around them.

There are numerous types of baby carriers available including wrap carriers (my personal favourite), ring slings, pouches, mei tais, soft structured carriers such as the Beco or Ergo, and framed back carriers. Each type of carrier has pros and cons. What's important is that you find one that works for you and your baby, one that you find easy to use and will use. You may find a local group or business where you can try a variety of carriers and learn how to use them properly and safely. A wonderful source of information on the internet about babywearing is the website www.thebabywearer.com. A very active and informative forum can be found on the site in addition to very helpful articles.

Responsive Parenting

"Attachment parenting" has become a common term over the past several years. Attachment parenting is centred around the goal of "forming and nurturing strong connections between parents and their children."[2] It highlights love, sensitivity, nurturing touch, proximity, positive discipline, and consistency. The term "attachment parenting" can sometimes have slightly negative connotations, bringing to mind a hippie-like mother who nurses constantly, co-sleeps, and carries her children everywhere. This is far from the truth. To avoid some of these connotations, I prefer the term "responsive parenting".

Responsive parenting simply means responding to the needs of your child and meeting their needs when they need them met. When you meet the need, the need will then go away. A newborn needs to have physical contact with its mother and quick attention given to its needs. Providing this intense attention does not create a needy child, but instead meets the need for attention and care allowing the child to develop independence and trust in those around them.

When breastfeeding hasn't worked out, one of the methods a mother has to meet the needs of her child has been removed, so ensuring responsiveness in other ways becomes even more important. Remember the biologically normal process of mothering. Think also of the normal process of lactation. Strive to meet the needs of your child in as biologically normal a manner as possible. This responsiveness will allow for a close relationship between you and your child and meet the needs of your baby, allowing him or her to develop independence and confidence in a loving relationship. Being responsive to your baby's needs will also make mothering easier. When our needs are met, not just as babies but throughout our lives, we are happier and more balanced people.

There Are Other Options

It is important to realize that there are other options available to you when breastfeeding doesn't work out as hoped. Other options you might consider include exclusively pumping[3], a combination of breastfeeding and pumping, partial breastfeeding with formula supplementation[4], donor milk[5], relactation[6], and formula feeding. Each option has its pros and cons. It is important that you consider all your options and also consider what each option means in terms of time commitment, cost, emotional impact, and effect on your family.

What is a mother?

In the end, being a mother is about being there for your child. It's about caring and nurturing and loving unconditionally. Being a mother means stepping up and taking responsibility, and also acknowledging our faults. None of us are perfect mothers. Personally, I have no interest in being a perfect mother. I am a flawed being, I admit—and I'm grateful for the grace that forgives me for my flaws. In the end, I am my children's mother because I'm there and I love them and I care for them—I would give my life for them. I soothe their hurts; I rock them after scary dreams; I discipline them when they stray too far from what is expected; I encourage their independence and individuality. This is what being a mother is all about. It's about having your heart walk around outside your body. What does being a mother mean to you? My guess is that if you really think about it, the way you nourish your infant will be only a small part of the equation.

In addition to what it means to be a mother, it's important to recognize the scope and timeline of motherhood. Motherhood will be an aspect of your life from the moment your first child is born until the day you die. Mothering doesn't end when your child becomes a teenager, or reaches the age of majority, or heads off to college, or gets married. You will be a mother for life. You will care about your children for your entire life. Your specific duties might change, but your overall role will never change. While breastfeeding is important and beneficial to a young child, it is only a small piece in the larger quilt of motherhood. If you do not achieve the breastfeeding relationship you had hoped for, start focusing on the other pieces of your quilt. With love and care, you will create a beautiful blanket of motherhood that will protect and care for your children for the rest of their lives.

≈≈≈

Cortney's Story

My personal attitude and feelings toward breastfeeding with my first baby leaned towards the idea that I was invincible; there was nothing that was going to stop me from feeding my babe. There was no "trying" about it. In fact, I was so convinced that it was going to work out fine for me that I never even considered what the alternative would be. I felt that any mom who was able to breastfeed and yet chose not to was skipping out on a very crucial experience for themselves and their child. It never even occurred to me to prepare for a situation in which I wasn't able to physically "perform the act" and never purchased any supplies. I was convinced it would just work out as "naturally" for me as everyone said it would.

I had planned on bottle-feeding my baby after I got breast-feeding well established, but I would be using breast milk, never formula! I had a bit of a negative attitude towards formula. I felt that formula was for moms that didn't want to give their babies the best start; it was a cop-out or something. I was certain that with the correct amount of patience and time, it would just...work. I was convinced of this by all of the material I had read and been told about breastfeeding in pre-natal classes, on baby related websites, and by doctors and nurses. There was a certain stigma attached to moms that didn't want to breastfeed, and I didn't want that association—I wanted to be in the "good books".

My plan, despite the discouragement I had encountered from many different health practitioners, was to get breastfeeding well established, establish a bond between my baby and me, and then begin to pump so that I would have some "freedom" from my babe. I also wanted to have my husband be able to share in the responsibility of feeding, as well as enjoy a close bond. I think that my expectation was that it would just work out that way, and again, nothing would stop me from doing this, regardless of the negative feedback I received from health practitioners. They gave me the impression that pumping and bottle-feeding was not the proper thing to do; I was to only feed directly from the breast at all times. I was determined to have things my way and have my freedom, so I kept focused on my idea and was deter-mined to do what I wanted.

I had intended to exclusively breastfeed for at least a good six months, introduce solids and continue to breastfeed as long as my baby wanted it. I really hadn't established a timeline for what I thought was right. I did know that I was not going to be breastfeeding a child that could actually ask for "boobie" or milk and pull up my shirt. I just couldn't see myself doing that! I never imagined that it would be as difficult as I experienced, nor did I think that it would not happen just as "naturally" as it was supposed to. I had assumed that there was a fair bit of work to get a supply established, and then it would all be easy peasy from there.

When my first babe arrived, we were sent home from the hospital with a clean bill of health for both my baby and myself, and I was told that a public health nurse would be in to check on us a day or two after discharge. We were told that breastfeeding was well on its way to working out well for us, and that we were just waiting for my milk supply to "arrive". My concern level was rising, however, every single time I fed my son because he had a huge appetite and I just couldn't seem to get him to fill up with colostrum. I kept getting the same answer over and over, though:"Your milk is just slow coming in and your latch is not great!" No one ever seemed to consider that there was an issue of any sort.

We had a horrible first night at home with a screaming baby—he was just so hungry. Being new parents, we had no idea why this child was not sleeping at all, and did not even think that hunger might be a cause as we had been told that we were getting enough into him with what supply I had. I called Tele-health (a provincial health information line) and the male nurse told me that I had to fix my latch and that there was nothing more he could help with. I was instructed to go see my family doc.

I called the hospital floor where we had been for the post-partum period. They told me I was no longer a patient and had to see my family doc. I called La Leche League, but received no answer from any of the representatives. I called the ER, no help there. I called the health unit in tears the next morning at 7:45

a.m. and they had a public health nurse at our door for 8:30 a.m. to help out. She checked our latch—it was horrible— and my nipples were in terrible shape. No consult was done in the hospital about this, and the nurses had kept telling me that my nipples had to toughen up. The health nurse that saw us weighed and assessed our son, determined that he had lost over 10% of his body weight from his discharge weight, and that we had to take action right then. She started us on an SNS (Supplemental Nursing System) with formula, a schedule for pumping after feeding the baby at the breast with the SNS, and told me she would be back to check on us the next day. I felt a little better, and my determination was still there to keep breastfeeding.

I really didn't sleep for the first two weeks after my son's birth because our schedule was to feed him at the breast with the SNS system, feed him with a bottle afterwards to top him up, then pump for twenty minutes on each breast, making sure that I did this rotation every two to three hours. I felt that I *had* to continue with it, because of my own drive, and because the whole medical field led me to believe that there simply was no excuse not to breastfeed. I was also told that this would definitely work to bring my supply in, and that it would only take a matter of a few weeks.

It never worked out. I never established any sort of supply at all, and we had to feed my son formula by bottle. I was so very disappointed that it didn't work out, but I was very lucky that I caught the weight loss and troubles early on so that we could make the switch to formula with no real issues for my son. I was hospitalized four weeks after I had my son with a gall bladder issue, liver troubles, and pancreas troubles and had to have multiple surgeries, so it worked out well that he was able to be independent of me to feed.

Moving into my second pregnancy, I assumed that there had to be something wrong with my first breastfeeding experience and that it would all work itself out. I was determined that I could get breastfeeding to work the second time around. I was well prepared to take all of the supplements, do some minor pumping to help with supply, investigate the issues further if it just didn't work out, and I got my information and supports organized to have a successful breastfeeding experience the second time. I had no idea of any physical conditions or issues that would prevent me from feeding or establishing a strong milk supply. Although I was interested in getting answers to the reasons why breastfeeding didn't work out with my son, I didn't receive any answers until after I had a second bad experience with my second child, my daughter.

When I was pregnant with my daughter, I was excited to try to breastfeed again. I was determined to make it work this time around and no issue was going to get in my way. I had lots of colostrum leaking while I was pregnant and was encouraged by this. My breasts really did not change much during pregnancy at all, but with the leaking, I was hopeful that things would change once my daughter was born. My midwives kept an eye on me and said there wasn't much we could do to ensure I established a strong milk supply while I was pregnant and I would have to wait until my baby was born.

When my daughter was born, I started off the same way I did with my son and I thought things would go okay. It was on the third night after her birth, while still in the hospital, that a nurse pointed out that my daughter, Brenna, was quite dry, and topped her up with a syringe of formula. Brenna was much happier and she settled well after that. The nurse was quite worried about the overall health of my baby and suggested that we establish a routine of feeding at breast and then syringe feeding with formula afterwards. My midwives agreed to this, and we kept up with it and also introduced cups for Brenna to lap from, SNS, and pumping with a hospital grade pump. I was given a referral to a local doctor who is also a lactation consultant and waited for that appointment while doing what we could to establish my supply—lots of pumping and a formula top-off with a syringe or cup. We continued along. I saw a nurse at Public Health who set me up with nipple shields, as my nipples were torn up and infected as they had been with my first baby, and made sure I had more details about the lactation consultant appointment.

When I got in to see the doctor, she examined me and watched me latch Brenna onto the breast for a feeding attempt. It was clear to her that I had an issue, and she was quick to give me a diagnosis of hypoplastic breasts, likely due to hormone issues relating to endometriosis, which I had been diagnosed with as a teenager. She told me there was never going to be any way that I could fully feed my baby, or future babies, at the breast and that I could maintain what I had for the time being as long as I wanted to. I was given a prescription for domperidone and continued taking a variety of supplements, pumping regularly, and supplementing with formula.

The diagnosis of hypoplastic breasts was harsh, and it was a real blow to me, but I knew that I *finally* had an answer. It didn't reduce the guilt, but I kept going and made sure that I was doing all I could to get the milk that I did have to my daughter. It was a minimal amount though, and I was very depressed and not happy with the prospect of continuing, but I did it because I thought it was best for my girl.

At eight weeks post-partum, when I brought my daughter to my breast, and she started screaming and refused to eat, I gave up. I took that as a sign that it was time to stop the torture of myself and of my daughter. I had already given up on pumping, but had continued with supplements, so I took them as long as I could, until I was certain this was the end. I continued feeding my daughter with formula in bottles after this point.

The experience, when I look back, was probably the hardest thing I have ever put myself through, and I still wonder if it was the right choice or not, with both babies. I feel sometimes that I did all that "stuff" to maintain any sort of breastfeeding on a selfish level, so that I could be the "perfect mom". I wanted so badly to provide the very best for my kids, and fought a brave, tough fight to make sure that I could do what I wanted. I was sure the second time around that I had it all organized and figured out, but when I received my diagnosis, it crushed my hopes. In some ways, I was happy to get the diagnosis, to help put answers to my questions, and to find out that there was a definitive reason why I couldn't feed my babes. I only wish I had someone tell me earlier on—perhaps when I was pregnant with my son, or just after he was born. I wanted to know earlier so I didn't have to put myself, my babies or my family through what we went through. I was happy to see that there was a reason, but sad at the same time.

After my son was born, along with issues from medical problems, I developed post-traumatic stress syndrome and depression, and I was convinced I was a failure. I got through it, worked with counsellors, and tried to get past the issue. I felt a tonne of guilt each time I gave my son a bottle, but it did get a little easier each time, and I continued to work past it, knowing that I would not let it happen to me again the second time.

When I was pregnant with my daughter, it brought back a lot of memories, and concerns as well. I was terrified to have the same issues with my daughter as I did with my son. I did not want to return to the same cycle of problems. When I again had breastfeeding challenges, this time with my daughter, I felt all of the pain from the first bad experience, and then again the guilt of not being able to make it work the second time around.

No one had ever mentioned to me that there was any possible reason why I couldn't breastfeed my son. Since he was okay on formula and I was okay after being in the hospital with all the other stuff going on, it was just left alone. This is a unfortunate part of this whole situation, really.

When I first got pregnant with my daughter, and I mean at the very beginning when I went to the doctor to get absolute confirmation that I was pregnant, I started asking if I could get help with figuring out what the problem may have been with my son that affecting breastfeeding. I asked if it was perhaps due to endometriosis, but my doctor and my nurse somewhat brushed that off and said that there was no way to determine a reason until I was further along in my pregnancy and my breast tissue started to develop again. I asked repeatedly and kept pushing, but got nowhere. I found it really frustrating that doctors and nurses don't mind telling you to breastfeed, but they don't really look into any problems that may be there, such as underlying conditions that may prevent proper development and affect milk supply. They brush it off for someone else to worry about, is how I see it.

I then got accepted into the midwives' practice at about two and a half months into my second pregnancy and started asking them if there were any reasons for the breastfeeding difficulties I experienced with my son. I was given basically the same answer. I asked if I could see a lactation consultant, but my midwives said there really wasn't much a lactation consultant could do until after the birth of my daughter. I never had anyone even physically examine me to see if there was any outward sugges-tion of concerns. One nurse guessed that hypoplastic breasts may be the reason, but it never came about to anything more than that.

I still feel sometimes that I have failed my children, but I am making my way through the grief of it all, and making sure that I don't beat myself up over it. I still feel sad when I think about the situation, and still have guilty pangs, but it gets easier every day.

I know that I never want to put myself through this again (we don't plan on anymore children), nor do I want to put my family through it. I still question why I did what I did and wonder if it was the right choice. I know that I will get through this experience, knowing I did what I could do, and that was the best there is. I know that my children will never look back on such a small fragment of their lives and say that I was horrible to them, or that it was wrong. I only want to move forward from now and share my story to help other moms that are out there so they don't have to go through what I went through.

I still feel that breastfeeding is the best for babies, moms, and the entire family unit, really. It is inexpensive, nutritionally superior, and an incredible way to bond with your babe. I will continue to promote breastfeeding to anyone who will listen. I do feel, however, that it is not for everyone, and it sometimes just won't work. I feel sad for moms that won't even try to feed their babies at the breast, but I have learned tolerance and know that I must respect their decisions, either way. I wish for more help and support for each mom and baby pair, both before and after birth. I feel that there simply isn't enough proper information, resources, support, and help for moms that are having anything but a "normal" experience with breastfeeding. I wish for more open-minded people, communities, health care, and society to help ease the burden with breastfeeding issues overall. I want to be able to help in any way that I can, to bring it out in the open that breastfeeding is not the only option, if you can't make it work it is okay, and that it is okay to feed your baby with formula. I know that if we ever did have another child, I would likely try to breastfeed with what I could, and then know formula was the way we had to go. But that will likely never happen, so it's a moot point!

Conclusion

"In the lap of the eternal spirit you have been nursed
and nurtured for ages."

Rabindranath Tagore

I have a friend who tried to breastfeed her first baby, made a
half-hearted effort for only a couple of days with her
second, and went straight to using formula with her third.
Her story isn't unique. I hear it all the time. Women who state, "I
tried breastfeeding my first child and it didn't work out. I'll just
feed formula. I'm not going to try *that* again." Why would
anyone want to try to breastfeed a second time? When you've
gone through the experience once and encountered pain, stress,
turmoil, frustration, and, quite possibly, anger, why would you
want to open yourself back up to that potential outcome?

For me, it was a deep, ingrained understanding that breastfeeding was what I was supposed to do as a mother. I don't
mean that in order to be a good mother you have to breastfeed.
No, I mean on a much deeper, biological, and perhaps even
spiritual level, breastfeeding just felt right to me. Can I attribute
this belief to my society, my culture? No. If anything my society
and culture kept whispering to me to give in to the pressures to
bottle-feed. But even though I endured a great deal of stress and
pain trying to breastfeed my first-born—and that ended in a

245

dismal failure—I still *needed* to breastfeed my daughter. Something in my very being craved the experience. And my guess is you likely feel the same way, which is why you are reading this book.

And really, should this be so surprising to us? We are, after all, mammals. We are biological beings given the ability to nourish our babies at our breasts. And yet, the fact that any of us want to try again still leaves me perplexed. What is it that drives us? And why does it not drive every woman? Why are some women so determined *not* to try again? I don't have the answers to that—although in this book I've attempted to present some of the influences that affect our decisions both to breastfeed and not to breastfeed—but I suspect a woman's decision, even adamant refusal, to breastfeed has a lot to do with societal influences and views on life.

The more I consider the question, and reflect on my own experience, I believe that the drive to breastfeed—aside from being a normal, biological expectation—is a desire for balance. From the moment we are born into this world, we have forces working against us that upset the inner, biological harmony of life. Our society and our biology are at odds, and all too often, society wins. Breastfeeding, to me, is a way to move the scale, even if just a bit, back towards biology—to take a step towards reconciling these two forces and ensuring it is not only my society having a say in how I mother my children.

When I was bottle-feeding my son, I remember the experience always being one of effort. It wasn't a time when I could relax and be a mother. It was another job to be done. I didn't like that feeling. Now, part of this might have had to do with the fact that I was exclusively pumping for my son, so time was at a premium and sitting to bottle-feed him was truly another twenty minutes that was added to the additional responsibilities of pumping and cleaning and sterilizing, on top of all the other tasks of mother-hood.

But nursing my daughter was a completely different exper-ience. Of course there were times when I was annoyed that she wanted to nurse *again* or that she was waking me for the third or fourth time in the night needing to nurse, but generally, my memories of nursing her are pleasant ones. They are moments of relaxation amid a hurried day, not a task to fit into an already busy schedule. Our regularly scheduled "quiet" time at the end of the day was an opportunity for the two of us to reconnect and relax before the busy dinner hour, and I missed that time after my daughter weaned. I always say that breastfeeding is a "lazy" way of mothering in the best sense of the word. It made feeding my child convenient and, after the initial few weeks of getting it all figured out, easy.

The desire we as women have to breastfeed still amazes me, but the understanding of what we gain from the experience of breastfeeding really does not. For me, amid all the chaos and confusion that motherhood can bring, moments of utter and profound peace have come through breastfeeding. There are images eternally etched into my memory of the quiet, calm moments nursing my daughter. And even though I ultimately was unable to breastfeed my son in the way I would have liked, there are still a couple of peaceful, endearing moments with my son that I'll cherish.

One such moment was when I was already well established as an exclusively pumping mom. I had accepted my fate and was no longer struggling to breastfeed. Yet, I would still see if he'd latch—just in case. One day he did, and with me sitting cross-legged on the floor and my son cradled at my breast, he un-latched and gave me the biggest, happiest smile ever. Just thinking about it now warms my heart and makes me realize that in the midst of all the pain, frustration, and heartache that surrounded our breastfeeding efforts, that one moment made it all worthwhile. Even if that one smile was all I ever got in terms of a breastfeeding connection, it was enough. And it perhaps is what made me so determined to try again the second time around. And I'm so glad I did.

Throughout the book we've covered a lot of ground. The biological basis of breastfeeding has been emphasized; the societal influences and medical interventions affecting breastfeeding have been investigated; the emotions surrounding breastfeeding have been discussed; and information to help you move forward into a new breastfeeding experience defining, and achieving, your own success has been presented. It is my hope that through this discussion you will have a renewed sense of faith in your body and an understanding of how to approach your next breastfeeding relationship. I also trust that you have had an opportunity to work through some of the lingering emotions from your first breastfeeding experience and have recognized what you did do in the face of a challenging situation.

Remember, you are an amazing mother! Your dedication to your baby—your desire to fully meet your baby's needs—is evidence of a deep yearning to do what you know is right, what is normal. *And you do know what is right for you and your baby.* Trust yourself; trust your body; trust your baby. Together you have the wisdom of generations. It is my sincere hope that you receive a breastfeeding relationship with your next baby that satisfies you and helps to heal the loss of your first breastfeeding experience, while at the same time helping you appreciate the gifts that came with it.

Acknowledgements

First and foremost I want to thank all the women who have communicated with me over the past several years and who have been so open and honest about their worries and emotions surrounding breastfeeding.

Thank you to the numerous women who generously shared their personal stories for this book and to those who encouraged me to write it. I hope that the end result meets with your approval and does justice to your experiences. You are all heroes!

Thank you to Michelle, Ying, and Sandy for reading an early version of the book and giving me such detailed and valuable feedback. Your experience, kindness, honesty, and knowledge mean so much.

Thank you to Sharon for editing the book. As an English teacher I know that every writer can benefit from a good editor, but until you stepped into the project I had no idea just how much a good editor can "impact" the written word. Thank you for your dedication and attention to detail.

Thank you to Diane for creating a beautiful cover that helps to express the deep emotions involved in breastfeeding and the close bond between a mother and her children, as well as the hope that comes with every new life we are gifted with.

Finally, I want to extend my gratitude to my family. Your support is what keeps me motivated and your love is what keeps me sane.

Breastfeeding, Take Two

Appendix

Establishing Breastfeeding and Overcoming Challenges

Key Elements to Establishing Breastfeeding

Importance of the First Feed

- Utilize the instincts a baby is born with.
- It is important to imprint early at the breast.
- Early feeding allows a baby to get an initial "dose" of colostrum and to regulate a baby's blood sugars.
- The first feed should ideally be within the first hour of birth and, if a baby is left to self-attach, will usually happen within this time period although birth interventions can impact a baby's first feeding.
- If the situation prevents the first feed from taking place within the first hour, a baby can still be allowed to self-attach. Plenty of skin-to-skin time is important to establishing breastfeeding.
- If latching difficulties persist, go back to the idea of self-attachment.

Baby-led/Mother Supported Latching

- Babies are born to latch and suckle; they are born with the reflexes and responses necessary to nurse.
- We merely need to allow it to happen and do not, in most cases, need to do anything but support the baby and follow her or his lead.
- Babies that are placed skin-to-skin between a mother's breasts can move, orient themselves to the breast (often the left side), and latch on by themselves with limited assistance.
- This type of baby-led latching can be continued as the nursing relationship develops.

Skin-to-Skin

- Maintains body temperature and regulates respiration. A light blanket over both the mother and baby is sufficient to maintain the baby's body temperature.
- Skin-to-skin contact between a mother and her baby allows for baby-led latching and should be continued throughout the first few days postpartum. A baby who has ample skin-to-skin contact will wake more frequently to nurse avoiding many common concerns in the early days.
- Skin-to-skin contact assists with bonding and boosts a mother's milk supply.

Crucial First 24-36 Hours

- Prolactin spikes in the immediate post-partum period and then quickly declines over the first 24-36 hours. It is important to nurse frequently during this time to utilize the boost of prolactin and establish the strongest milk supply possible.

- Keeping your baby close during this time and nursing frequently provides the baby with important colostrum prior to the increase in milk production.
- The prolactin receptor theory suggests that frequent stimulation during the early hours and days sets long-term milk production.

Importance of Rooming-In and Close Proximity of Mother and Baby

- Rooming-in allows for a baby to have frequent access to the breast and for a mother to respond quickly to hunger cues.
- It also removes the possibility of hospital staff giving bottles/supplement without permission.
- Consider having your baby co-sleep if it is safe to do so and allow for as much skin-to-skin contact as possible.

Delaying Routine Procedures

- Allows baby to act on instinct to locate breast and latch and to gain the benefits of colostrum as soon as possible.
- Delaying routine procedures helps to ensure the baby is not traumatized and does not go into a parasympathetic state where a baby will withdraw and conserve thereby making breastfeeding more challenging.
- Trauma can put a baby into a deep sleep which is difficult to wake them from.

Delaying First Bath

- An initial bath, especially immediately after delivery, can be traumatizing to a newborn and can lead to difficulties for the baby maintaining body temperature.
- Smell is a very important sense for newborns and a baby seems to utilize the scent of the amniotic fluid on their hands to locate the nipple
- If your baby has been cleaned prior to their first attempt to latch, try to leave their hands alone and do not wash.

Dangers of Giving Formula/Using Bottles/Pacifiers

- Even one feeding of formula changes a baby's gut flora and it takes a long time to return to normal.
- Supplementation can interfere with a mother's initiation and maintenance of her milk supply.
- Using artificial nipples and/or pacifiers can interfere with baby's suck and/or lead to nipple preference. Babies do not suckle on an artificial nipple in the same way as at their mother's breast.
- Pacifiers can mask hunger cues and cause a baby to miss needed feedings thereby reducing the stimulation to mom and causing a reduction in milk supply. Pacifiers may not be the cause of early weaning in and of themselves, but their use may indicate breastfeeding problems.[1]

Frequency of Feeds

- Frequent nursing is important for milk production and for fat transfer.

- Allowing a baby to nurse on "demand" takes into account the variation in storage capacity between women and the variation in intake requirements between babies.
- Trying to schedule a baby's feeding is detrimental to a mother's milk supply and works against a baby's natural rhythms.

How do you know if your baby is getting enough milk?

Input=Output—Watching Diapers
- Typically one wet/dirty diaper per day of life for the first three days of life.
- After day four, baby should have at least three to four stooled diapers daily (size of a quarter or larger) and stools should be yellow; prior to this, stool will transition from black meconium through to the yellow stool.
- Normal stool of a breastfed babe is soft and sometimes seedy or like curd.
- Colour of stool can vary: green, orange, yellow are all normal variations although green stool in combination with excessive gas, pain, or poor weight gain can be a signal of difficulties.
- After about four weeks, stooling patterns may change. Some breastfed babies do not have frequent bowel movements and may go as long as seven or more days between dirty diapers. As long as stool is still loose and weight gain is good, this isn't a cause for concern.
- Once milk supply has increased, five to six wet diapers/day.

- It can be difficult to determine just how wet a diaper is. Try pouring about three tablespoons of water into a clean diaper to feel how wet that is for comparison.
- Put a tissue in the diaper, to see when it has been wetted or use cloth diapers.
- As baby grows, wet diapers may decrease slightly but amounts will stay consistent as the bladder's capacity increases.

Weight Gain

- May lose up to 7% of weight in the first few days. 10% is a caution flag and breastfeeding needs to be evaluated, however…
- Babies whose mothers were on IV fluids during delivery may have excess fluids to excrete and this may cause a misleading decrease in weight in the early days of life.
- Baby should regain birth weight by ten days.
- The average breastfed newborn gains around 5-7 ounces/week (170 grams/week). Anywhere from 0.5 to 1 ounce/day or 15-30 grams/day—or more!
- Weight gain typically slows after about three months to 4-5 ounces/week (113-142 grams/week) and again around six months of age to about 2-4 ounces/week (57-113 grams/week).
- Ensure your doctor is using the most recent WHO growth charts that are based on the biologically normal growth patterns of a breastfed baby! Weight gain patterns vary significantly between breastfed and formula-fed babes—or use the charts yourself.

Suck-Pause-Swallow

- Initial suckling pattern to elicit let-down is rapid, short sucks which will stimulate a let-down.
- Suckling pattern of active nursing—suck, pause as the chin drops and mouth fills with milk, swallow; suckling is long draws and slower than the initial suckling to elicit let-down.
- Should have an extended length of active suckling with brief pauses.
- Baby will return to quick, initial suckling pattern to elicit additional let-downs since oxytocin is released in waves.

Audible/Visible Swallowing

- "Caw-caw-caw" sound as baby swallows.
- You should hear swallowing when the milk flow is strong.
- Most importantly, you should see the chin drop and throat swallow. You will see deep jaw excursions as the jaw drops to swallow a mouthful of milk.

Breasts Should Soften After a Nursing Session

- This is useful in the early days and first few weeks of nursing, but once your milk supply regulates and the autocrine control takes over, you will not have the same fullness in your breasts before a feeding. This is completely normal and usually happens around four weeks post-partum.

Is your baby content? Not a good trustworthy gauge of how breastfeeding is going.

- Some babies who are not nursing effectively will become lethargic and seem like a "good" baby.
- While we all want a content baby, do not rely on this indicator alone to determine how breastfeeding is going.
- A baby who is not content may have various other problems that would not necessarily be improved by early weaning.

Is your baby sleeping well? Not a reliable indicator of breastfeeding success.

- Lack of calories can cause babies to conserve what energy they do have.
- Sleep is the best way to conserve energy.
- This can be a survival tactic for babies who are not breastfeeding well.
- Ensure your baby is nursing well, transferring milk, has plenty of wet/dirty diapers, gaining weight.
- Get assessment by a LC if there is indication of concern.
- If all the other indicators suggest things are going well, then consider yourself lucky to have a baby who sleeps well.

Overcoming Challenges

Engorgement

- Ensure baby is latching well and nursing effectively.
- If baby isn't nursing well, express frequently.
- Nurse frequently and empty breasts as fully as possible.
- You can use ibuprofen or acetaminophen for discomfort.
- Use cold packs in between feedings and warm, moist compresses just prior to feeding (do not use warm for more than a few minutes).
- For an effective cold pack, pour some water in a newborn disposable diaper. Shape the diaper into a u-shape and put it in the freezer to get cold. Use a cloth or towel between the diaper and breast.
- Use massage prior to nursing.
- Use breast compressions while nursing. Firm, consistent pressure and firm circular massage can assist in releasing ducts and emptying more fully.
- If your baby is having difficulty latching, hand express or use breast pump to remove some milk and soften your breasts and areolas prior to nursing.
- Cabbage leaves have been anecdotally reported as being helpful. Use cold, crushed green cabbage leaves and place around your breasts in your bra (not on nipple) and leave until wilted. Do not overuse as they also have been reported to reduce milk supply.

- Wear a supportive bra 24 hours a day but do not wear underwires or anything that is too constricting.
- Engorgement will normally subside within 12-48 hours if properly treated.

Non-Latching Baby

- Get help from a breastfeeding professional if possible.
- It is paramount to feed the baby and you may need to use alternative feeding strategies such as a supplemental nursing system, cup, or syringe.
- Maintain your milk supply; get a hospital grade pump and pump 8+ times/day for approximately 15-20 minutes/session.
- Have lots of skin-to-skin contact; take your baby to bed skin-to-skin and just spend time with your baby; bathe with your baby; practice kangaroo care; and wear your baby in a sling or wrap.
- Allow baby to take the lead and self-latch. Follow the baby-led latching guidelines and allow your baby to set the pace and use his or her instincts.
- Be patient and stop a session if you or baby gets upset.

Delayed Lactogenesis II

- Understand that certain labour interventions or health conditions (e.g. diabetes, PCOS) can impact the onset of lactogenesis II; even smoking and obesity can reduce prolactin levels and impact milk supply.

- First thing is to feed the baby. It is preferable to use a feeding method other than a bottle if possible to avoid the possibility of nipple preference.
- Allow your baby free access to the breast and nurse as often as possible.
- Use a breast pump to ensure you are receiving sufficient stimulation.
- Be persistent and patient. Supply will usually increase by 7-10 days.
- If supply does not increase, seek the advice of lactation professional and return to your doctor for an examination.

Sore Nipples

- Determine the cause of the soreness if at all possible.
- Fix the latch if there is a problem with latch; and optimize the latch.
- Have the baby's oral anatomy assessed if pain does not go away and you feel the latch is good.
- Use lanolin to aid in healing and keep nipples moist, although use caution if you suspect you might have a yeast infection.
- May consider using hydrogels to promote moist wound healing.
- Many moms experience some soreness or discomfort over the first few days of breastfeeding; this should resolve after a week or two. Discomfort usually is only at the point of the baby initially latching on and usually subsides during a feeding.

- If soreness doesn't get better, gets worse, or if nipples become cracked, bleeding, or damaged, seek help!

Nipple Preference/Confusion

- Best way to avoid nipple preference/confusion is by avoiding the use of artificial nipples or pacifiers until your baby is nursing very well and your milk supply is well established — usually around four weeks.
- Nipple preference is largely an issue of flow rate; bottles deliver milk at a much faster rate and some babies get used to the ease of the bottle and begin to expect the fast flow.
- Encourage your baby to be at breast with lots of skin-to-skin time and snuggles.
- Remember breastfeeding is not just about nourishment.
- If you are using artificial nipples, use a slow flow nipple.

Yeast

- Antibiotics can make you more susceptible to a yeast infection.
- Nipple or breast pain after a period of pain-free nursing may indicate yeast.
- Symptoms of a yeast infection include nipple/areola redness, shininess, itchiness, pain, burning pain that gets worse through nursing sessions, and pain in between nursing sessions.
- Babies can also get a yeast infection (thrush) in the mouth or diaper area.

- There are a number of natural remedies that are sometimes suggested for yeast, but they are outside of the scope of this book to discuss. Certainly do some research.
- Your doctor can prescribe antifungal medications for you and your baby if necessary. See a lactation consultant or your doctor.
- Wash everything that comes in contact with your breasts in hot water. Change breast pads regularly and wash your bras daily.
- Yeast is naturally occurring in our bodies. A yeast infection is more accurately a yeast overgrowth. Dietary and lifestyles changes may be necessary to truly bring a balance back to your body.
- Also consider naturopathic or homeopathic treatments.

Blocked Duct

- Blocked ducts are indicated by one or more of the following: a red spot on the breast, a hot spot on the breast, an area that is sore or painful, a lump or hard spot that can be felt in the breast.
- Use massage while nursing your baby, hot moist compresses prior to nursing, and compressions while nursing to work out the blockage in the ducts and clear out the milk.
- You may try to position your baby with his or her chin pointing towards the blockage although this isn't always practical.
- Nurse frequently and empty your breasts as fully as possible.
- Avoid wearing tight bras or underwire bras.

- Blocked ducts usually resolve within 24 hours or so. If yours does not, or if it is accompanied by fever, chills, soreness, or other symptoms of illness, see your doctor to rule out anything more serious.

Mastitis

- Mastitis is an infection in the breast.
- A breast infection can be a result of unresolved blocked ducts or nipple trauma but this is not always the case.
- Symptoms can include fever, a feeling of being unwell, flu symptoms, a hot red spot on the breast, and localized or generalized soreness.
- Mastitis can resolve spontaneously—usually within 24 hours—but if it worsens, is no better after 12-24 hours, or if you are extremely ill, you will require a prescription for antibiotics from your doctor.
- Do *not* stop nursing! There is no reason to quit nursing because of mastitis. You must continue to remove the milk in your breasts or the infection could worsen.
- Increase your fluid intake and take baby to bed and rest.

Sleepy Baby

- If you have a sleepy baby, ensure the baby's latch is good and that the baby is transferring milk; the baby may be sleepy because he or she is not eating enough.
- When nursing, switch breasts as soon as your baby starts to lose interest and continue to

"switch nurse" until you can no longer maintain nursing.

- Undress your baby to the diaper before nursing.
- Use skin-to-skin contact to encourage the baby's instinctive behaviours.
- Dim the lights; sometimes babies will keep their eyes closed if it is too bright.
- Use the "doll eyes" technique of gently laying down and sitting up the baby as you would a doll to open and close their eyes.
- Increase your baby's stimulation by rubbing her back in circular motions, rubbing the scalp, rubbing hands and feet, and bicycling her legs.
- Change your baby's diaper before offering the other breast to wake the baby up a bit.
- Monitor your baby's output and weight gain closely to ensure sufficient milk intake.
- Work with a lactation consultant or specialist to overcome the underlying issues that may be causing your baby to be excessively sleepy.

Breastfeeding, Take Two

Endnotes and References

Chapter 1- The Great Balancing Act

1. Katherine Dettwyler, "A Natural Age of Weaning," *Thoughts on Breastfeeding,* www.kathydettwyler.org

2. B. Chalmers, C. Levitt, M. Heaman, B.O'Brien, R. Sauve, J. Kaczorowski. "Breastfeeding rates and hospital breastfeeding practices in Canada: a national survey of women." *Birth.* Vol. 36, No. 2 (June 2009): 122-32.

3. Katherine Dettwyler, "A Natural Age of Weaning," *Thoughts on Breastfeeding,* www.kathydettwyler.org

4. Jean Liedloff, *The Continuum Concept.* (Cambridge: Perseus Books, 1977), 24.

5. For a short, eye-opening video related to self-attachment see *Delivery Self-Attachment* by Dr. Lennart Righard and Margaret Alade.

6. Ruth Feldman, "Evidence for a Neuroendocrinological Foundation of Human Affiliation: Plasma Oxytocin Levels Across Pregnancy and the Postpartum Period Predict Mother-Infant Bonding," *Psychological Science*, Vol. 18, No. 11 (November 2007): 965-970.

7. Karen Bales, "Oxytocin has Dose-dependent Developmental Effects on Pair-bonding and Alloparental Care in Female Prairie Voles," *Hormones and Behavior*, Vol. 52, No. 2 (2007): 272-279.

8. Elizabeth Sibolboro Mezzacappa, "Breastfeeding and Maternal Stress Response and Health," *Nutrition Reviews*, Vol. 62, No. 7 (July 2004): 261-268.

9. Maureen Wimberly Groer et al., "Postpartum Stress: Current Concepts and the Possible Protective Role of Breast-

feeding," *Journal of Obstetric, Gynecologic, and Neonatal Nursing,* Vol. 31, No. 4 *(July/August 2001)*: 411-417.

10. Alison Stuebe, *"Does breastfeeding prevent postpartum depression?"* Breastfeeding Medicine Blog, www.bfmed. wordpress.com

11. Alison Stuebe, *"Does breastfeeding prevent postpartum depression?"*

12. Center for Disease Control, "Breastfeeding Report Card, United States: Outcome Indicators," www.cdc.gov/ breastfeeding/data/reportcard2.htm

13. Statistics Canada, "Breastfeeding, 2009," www.statcan. gc.ca/pub/82-625-x/2010002/article/11269-eng.htm

Chapter 2- What's Society Got to Do With It?

1. Cynthia Good Mojab, "The Cultural Art of Breastfeeding," Leaven, Vol. 36, No. 5 (Oct./Nov. 2000): 87-91.

2. Julia Glass, "The Whole Truth (and Nothing but the Truth)" in *Unbuttoned: Women Open Up About the Pleasures, Pains, and Politics of Breastfeeding,* ed. Dana Sullivan and Maureen Connolly (Boston: The Harvard Common Press, 2009), 8.

3. It's not my intention to provide a deep investigation into the history of breastfeeding, the rise of infant formula, or the social and political issues surrounding breastfeeding, but if you're interested there are a number of excellent books on the subject including *The Politics of Breastfeeding* by Gabrielle Palmer; *Mother's Milk* by Bernice Hausman; and *Milk, Money, and Madness* by Naomi Baumslag.

4. Samir Arora, Cheryl McJunkin, Julie Wehrer, and Phyllis Kuhn, "Major Factors Influencing Breastfeeding Rates: Mother's Perception of Father's Breastfeeding Attitude and Milk Supply," *Pediatrics,* Vol. 106, No. 5 (November 2000): e67.

5. Diane Wiessinger, "What About Dad?" Common Sense Breastfeeding, www.normalfed.com/Why/dad.html

6. My OB Said What, http://myobsaidwhat.com

7. Sarah Seltzer, "'Twilight Sleep': Is the Past Prologue for Today's Debates Over Birthing Choices?" RH Reality Check, http://www.rhrealitycheck.org/blog/2009/09/29/twilight-sleep-is-the-past-prologue-todays-debates-over-birthing-choices

8. For an interesting view on modern pregnancy and childbirth see the film *The Business of Being Born* and the soon to be released *One World Birth*.

9. *Sesame Street,* "Buffy nurses Cody," http://www.youtube.com/watch?v=7-L-Fg7lWgQ (accessed January 28, 2011).

10. Cynthia Good Mojab, "Unexpected mothering," Ammawell, http://home.comcast.net/~ammawell/expectations.html

Chapter 3- The Unknown "Why"

1. For information on breastfeeding rates see the Center for Disease Control, "Breastfeeding Report Card, United States: Outcome Indicators," www.cdc.gov/breastfeeding/data/reportcard2 and Statistics Canada, "Breastfeeding, 2009," www.statcan.gc.ca/pub/82-625-x/2010002/article/11269-eng.htm as well as Childinfo, http://www.childinfo.org/breastfeeding_countrydata.php.

2. Dr. Michelle Gibson, interviewed Kingston, Ontario, May 21, 2011.

3. ibid.

4. Sandy Stevenson, email message to author, July 9, 2011.

5. Judith Gutowski, comment posted on LactNew, July 7, 2011. Used with permission.

6. ibid.

7. Sandy Stevenson, email message to author, July 9, 2011.

8. *Global Strategy on Infant and Young Child Feeding,* World Health Organization, 2003. http://whqlibdoc.who.int/publications/2003/9241562218.pdf

9. For information on exclusively pumping see www.exclusivelypumping.com.

10. Ina May Gaskin, *Ina May's Guide to Childbirth* (New York: Bantam Dell, 2003), 141-142.

11. Canadian Institute for Health Information, "Primary Caesarean Section Rates, by province and territory," http://www.cihi.ca/CIHI-ext-portal/internet/en/document/health+system+performance/indicators/performance/release_1 6dec10_fig3 (accessed June 10, 2011) and "Births: Preliminary Data for 2007,"*National Vital Statistics Report,* http://www.cdc.gov/nchs/data/nvsr/nvsr57/nvsr57_12.pdf

12. Naomi Bromberg Bar-Yam, "Fathers and Breastfeeding: A Review of the Literature," *Journal of Human Lactation,* Vol. 13, No. 1 (March 1997): 45-50.

Chapter 4- Do You Think I'm Guilty?

1. Diane Wiessinger, "Watch Your Language," *Journal of Human Lactation*, Vol. 12, No. 1 (1996): 1-4.

2. Gina Crosley Corcoran, "When It Comes to Breastfeeding We Can't Handle the Truth," *The Feminist Breeder*, http://thefeministbreeder.com/when-it-comes-to-breastfeeding-we-cant-handle-the-truth

3. "Births: Preliminary Data for 2007,"*National Vital Statistics Report.*

4. Jessica Restaino, "Drained" in *Unbuttoned: Women Open Up About the Pleasures, Pains, and Politics of Breastfeeding*, ed. Dana Sullivan and Maureen Connolly (Boston: The Harvard Common Press, 2009), 146.

5. Jessica Restaino, "Drained" in *Unbuttoned: Women Open Up About the Pleasures, Pains, and Politics of Breastfeeding,* 148.

6. Jessica Restaino, "Drained" in *Unbuttoned: Women Open Up About the Pleasures, Pains, and Politics of Breastfeeding,* 146.

7. "intentions," Merriam-Webster.com, http://www.merriam-webster.com/dictionary/intentions

Chapter 5- The Best-Laid Plans

1. La Leche League International, "What is colostrum? How does it benefit my baby?" La Leche League International, http://www.llli.org/FAQ/colostrum.html

Chapter 6- An Experience By Any Other Name...

1. Jennifer Restaino, "Drained" in *Unbuttoned: Women Open Up About the Pleasures, Pains, and Politics of Breastfeeding,* ed. Dana Sullivan and Maureen Connolly (Boston: The Harvard Common Press, 2009), 149-150.

2. Paula Spencer, "Step One, Try It; Step Two, Whatever Works" in *Unbuttoned: Women Open Up About the Pleasures, Pains, and Politics of Breastfeeding,* ed. Dana Sullivan and Maureen Connolly (Boston: The Harvard Common Press, 2009), 66.

Chapter 7- Let's Get Back to Basics

1. Cynthia Good Mojab, "The Cultural Art of Breastfeeding,"*Leaven*, Vol. 36, No. 5 (2000): 87-91.

2. Marsha Walker, "Just One Bottle Won't Hurt—Or Will It?" National Alliance for Breastfeeding Advocacy, http://www.naba-breastfeeding.org/images/Just%20One %20Bottle.pdf

3. Peter E. Hartmann, Robyn A. Owens, David B. Cox, *and* Jacqueline C. Kent, *"Breast Development and Control of Milk Synthesis," Food and Nutrition Bulletin,* Vol. 17, No. 4 (December 1996), http://archive.unu.edu/unupress/food/8F174e/ 8F174E02.htm

4. Kelly Bonyata, "How does milk production work?" Kelly-mom, http://www.kellymom.com/bf/supply/milk

production.htm

5. Jacqueline Kent, Leon Mitoulas, Mark Cregan, Donna Ramsay, Dorota Doherty, Peter Hartman, "Volume and Frequency of Breastfeedings and Fat Content of Breast Milk Throughout the Day," *Pediatrics*, Vol. 117, No. 3 (March 2006): e387-e395.

6. See Jean Liedloff's *Continuum Concept* for further discussion on this idea.

7. Nancy Mohrbacher and Kathleen Kendall-Tackett, *Breastfeeding Made Simple* (Oakland: New Harbinger Publications, 2005).

8. Mary Kroeger with Linda J. Smith, *Impact of Birthing Practices on Breastfeeding* (Sudbury: Jones and Barlett, 2004), 98.

9. Judith Gutowski, comment posted on LactNew, July 7, 2011. Used with permission.

10. Michel Odent, "Drips of Synthetic Oxytocin, " Womb Ecology, http://wombecology.com/oxytocin.html (accessed November 2, 2010).

11. Siranda Torvaldsen, Christine L. Roberts, Judy M. Simpson, Jane F. Thompson, and David A. Ellwood, "Intrapartum epidural analgesia and breastfeeding: a prospective cohort study," *International Breastfeeding Journal,* Vol. 1, No. 24 (December 2006), accessed online http://www.international breastfeedingjournal.com/content/1/1/24.

12. Jan Riordan, "Epidurals and Breastfeeding," *Breastfeeding Abstracts*, Vol. 19, No. 2 (November 1999): 11-12.

13. Dennis J. Baumgarder, Patricia Muehl, Mary Fischer, and Bridget Pribbenow, "Effect of Labor Epidural Anesthesia on Breast-Feeding of Healthy Full-Term Newborns Delivered Vaginally," *Journal of American Board of Family Medicine*, Vol. 16, No. 1 (2003).

14. Pamela Hill, Sharron Humenick, Mary Brennan, and Deborah Wooley, "Does Early Supplementation Affect Long-

Term Breastfeeding?" *Clinical Pediatrics*, Vol. 36, No. 6 (June 1997): 345-350.

15. Breastfeeding Committee for Canada, "Guidelines for WHO/UNICEF Baby-Friendly Initiative in Canada: The Ten Steps and Practice Outcome Indicators for Baby Friendly Hospitals," March 24, 2004, www.breastfeedingcanada.ca.

16. Mary Kroeger with Linda J. Smith, *Impact of Birthing Practices on Breastfeeding*, 98.

17. Mary Kroeger with Linda J. Smith, *Impact of Birthing Practices on Breastfeeding*, 184.

18. Mary Kroeger with Linda J. Smith, *Impact of Birthing Practices on Breastfeeding*, 189.

19. For further information about Kangaroo Mother Care see Dr. Nils Berman's website at www.kangaroomothercare.com.

20. Meredith Small, Professor of Anthropology, Cornell University quoted in http://indiana.academia.edu/BridgetMcGann/Talks/30027/Why_Babies_Cry_The_Evolutionary_Origins_of_Infant_Communication

21. For further discussion of how this division between our biology and society affects parenting see "Colic: A Culture Bound Syndrome" by Bridget McGann, http://Indiana .academia.edu/BridgetMcGann/Papers/589744/Colic_A_Culture-Bound_Syndrome.

22. See www.thebabywearer.com for more information on babywearing.

23. Cecilia Jevitt, Ivonne Hernandez, Maureen Groër, "Lactation Complicated by Overweight and Obesity: Supporting the Mother and Newborn," *Journal of Midwifery and Women's Health*, Vol. 52, No.6 (2007): 606-613.

24. Nancy M. Hurst, "Recognizing and Treating Delayed or Failed Lactogenesis II ,"*Journal of Midwifery and Women's Health*, Vol. 52, No. 6 (2007): 588-594.

25. Nancy M. Hurst, "Recognizing and Treating Delayed or Failed Lactogenesis II ,"*Journal of Midwifery and Women's Health.*

26. Jihong Liu, Kenneth D. Rosenberg, Alfredo P. Sandoval, "Breastfeeding Duration and Perinatal Cigarette Smoking," *American Journal of Public Health*, Vol. 96, No. 2 (2006): 309-314.

27. K.F. Ilett, T.W. Hale, M. Page-Sharp, J.H. Kristensen, R. Kohan , and L.P. Hackett, "Use of Nicotine Patches in Breast-Feeding Mothers: Transfer of Nicotine and Cotinine Into Human Milk," *Clinical Pharmacology Therapeutics*, Vol. 74 (2003): 516-524.

28. L. Batstra , M. Hadders-Algra , and J. Neeleman , "Effect of Antenatal Exposure to Maternal Smoking on Behavioral Problems and Academic Achievement in Childhood: Prospective Evidence From a Dutch Birth Cohort" *Early Human Development,* Volume 75 (2003): 21-33.

29. J.J. Jaakkola and M. Gissler, "Maternal Smoking in Pregnancy, Fetal Development, and Childhood Asthma," *American Journal of Public Health*, Vol. 94 (2004): 136-140.

30. H. Sawnani , T. Jackson, T. Murphy, R. Beckerman , N. Simakajornboon, "The Effect of Maternal Smoking on Respiratory and Arousal Patterns in Preterm Infants During Sleep," *American Journal of Respiratory and Critical Care Medicine* (December 2003).

31. Jan Riordan, *Breastfeeding and Human Lactation* (Sudbury: Jones and Bartlett 2005), 483.

32. Nancy Howat and Hilary Jacobson, "Polycystic Ovarian Syndrome (PCOS) and Breastfeeding," MOBI Motherhood International, http://www.mobimotherhood.org/MM/article-pcos.aspx.

33. Kelly Bonyata, "Breastfeeding and Polycystic Ovarian Syndrome, "Kellymom, http://www.kellymom.com/bf/concerns/mom/pcos.html.

34. See *Making More Milk* by Diane West and Lisa Marasco for information on increasing milk supply and possible methods of lactation management for women with PCOS.
35. For a visual description of hypoplastic breasts see the website www.007b.com.

Chapter 8- Create Your Experience

1. For information about the fourth trimester see *The Happiest Baby on the Block* by Dr. Harvey Karp.
2. Heidi Raykeil, "Breast-laid Plans," in *Unbuttoned: Women Open Up About the Pleasures, Pains, and Politics of Breastfeeding*, ed. Dana Sullivan and Maureen Connolly (Boston: The Harvard Common Press, 2009), 41.
3. To find a lactation consultant in your area visit the International Lactation Consultants Association website at www.ilca.org.
4. www.biologicalnurturing.com
5. ibid.
6. Mari Douma, "Baby-led Latching: An 'intuitive' approach to learning how to breastfeed," *Ontario Breastfeeding Committee Newsletter*, Vol. 4, No. 4 (Dec. 2005): 2-3.

Chapter 9- And If It Should Happen Again?

1. Dee Kassing, "Bottle-feeding as a Tool to Reinforce Breast-feeding," *The Journal of Human Lactation*, Vol. 18, No. 1 (Feb. 2002): 56-60.
2. Attachment Parenting International, "What is API All About?," http://www.attachmentparenting.org /principles/principles.php.
3. For information about the option of exclusively pumping see *Exclusively Pumping Breast Milk: A Guide to Providing Expressed Breast Milk for Your Baby* by Stephanie Casemore and the website www.exclusivelypumping.com.

4. For information on combining breastfeeding and bottle-feeding see *Balancing Breast and Bottle* by Amy Peterson.
5. For information on milk banks see the Human Milk Banking Association of North America's website www.hmbana.org.
6. For information on relactation see the WHO publication "Relactation: review of experience and recommendations for practice," http://www.who.int/child_adolescent_health /documents/who_chs_cah_98_14/en/index.html.

Appendix
1. Sumi Sexton, MD, and Ruby Natale, PhD, PysD, "Risks and Benefits of Pacifiers," *American Family Physician*, Vol. 15, No. 8 (April 15 2009): 681-685.

Index

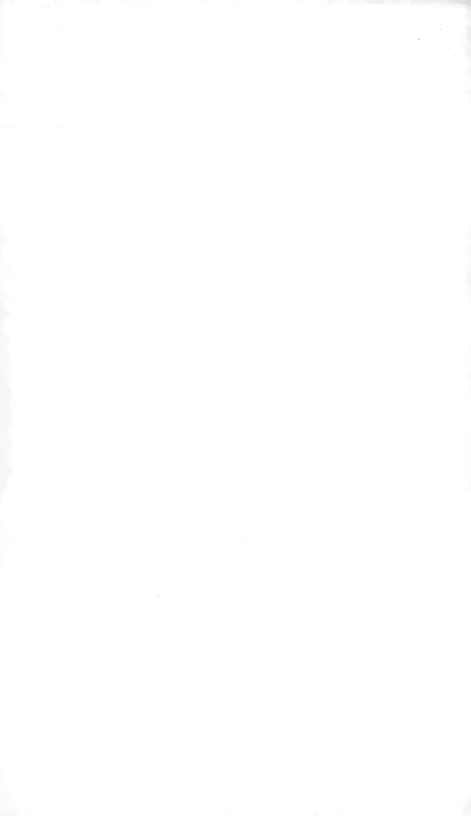

Lightning Source UK Ltd.
Milton Keynes UK
UKHW022301141220
375052UK00010B/992